# The Foundations of Shiatsu

**Chris Jarmey**

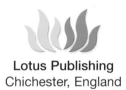

**Lotus Publishing**
Chichester, England

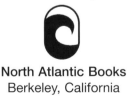

**North Atlantic Books**
Berkeley, California

First published in 2007 by
**Lotus Publishing**
3. Chapel Street, Chichester, PO19 1BU and
**North Atlantic Books**
P O Box 12327
Berkeley, California 94712

**Photographs** Doralba Picerno
**Illustrations** Michael Evdemon, Yiannis Tiropolis
**Models** Tom Hawthorn, Shampa Rahman, Patricia Leeson
**Text Design** Wendy Craig
**Cover Design** Wendy Craig
**Printed and Bound** in the UK by The Bath Press

**The Foundations of Shiatsu** is sponsored by the Society for the Study of Native Arts and Sciences, a non-profit educational corporation whose goals are to develop an educational and cross-cultural perspective linking various scientific, social, and artistic fields; to nurture a holistic view of arts, sciences, humanities, and healing; and to publish and distribute literature on the relationship of mind, body, and nature.

**British Library Cataloguing in Publication Data**
A CIP record for this book is available from the British Library
ISBN 978 1 905367 05 4 (Lotus Publishing)
ISBN 978 1 55643 639 0 (North Atlantic Books)

**Library of Congress Cataloguing-in-Publication Data**
Jarmey, Chris.
 The foundations of shiatsu / Chris Jarmey.
    p. ; cm.
 Includes bibliographical references and index.
  ISBN 978-1-905367-05-4 (pbk. : Lotus Pub.) -- ISBN 978-1-55643-639-0 (pbk.
: North Atlantic Books)
 1. Acupressure.  I. Title.
 [DNLM: 1. Acupressure--methods.  WB 369.5.A17 J37f 2007]
RM723.A27J372 2007
615.8'22--dc22
                                                            2007001993

# Contents

# Useful addresses

As there are many shiatsu schools worldwide, it is difficult to recommend individual schools. So it is suggested that you contact the relevant governing body within your country via their website, to find a suitable local school in your area. The only school listed is that of the author, who offers a full and comprehensive training through his network of schools.

**Australia**

www.staa.org.au/

**New Zealand**

www.spaanz.kiwinz.net/

**Europe**

www.shiatsu-esf.org/

**The European Shiatsu School**

Branches throughout the UK, Eire, Greece and Spain
Central administration: Highbank, Lockeridge, Marlborough, SN8 4EQ, UK
Tel.: 0845 166 5144
www.shiatsu.net

**United Kingdom**

www.shiatsusociety.org/

**USA**

www.aobta.org/

# Introduction

If you had asked a random selection of European, American or Australasian lay persons in 1975 the question, "what is shiatsu?", the reply would almost certainly have been, "I have no idea!" If you had asked them in 1985, most would have given the same answer, whilst a few would have described it as something similar to acupuncture but without needles. By 1995, public awareness had grown considerably. Significant numbers were actually studying its basic techniques. In fact between 1985 and 1995 shiatsu had experienced a rapid increase in popularity, greater than the growth of interest in complementary healing methods generally. Why this should be so is most likely due to the fact that many more people are not only seeking alternative methods to combat disease and remain healthy; they are also looking for some sort of inner meaning and purpose to their lives.

So, what is shiatsu, and how does it fulfil the dual role of a healing system and a method for personal development? Perhaps it is easier to first discuss what it is not. It is not merely acupuncture without needles or acupressure, although acupressure can be considered a sub-division of shiatsu. Neither is it simply an oriental method of physiotherapy or soft tissue manipulation; although if assessed purely from its range of physical techniques, it does incorporate aspects of these methods.

The fundamental principle of shiatsu is to hold, with clear mental focus, sustained stationary contact with a receiving person's body using thumbs, fingers, palms or sometimes elbows or knees; with sufficient patience to wait for a response in the receiver's subtle energy or Ki (qi, ch'i) flow. A variety of stretching, rotating and levering techniques may be required to reduce the receiver's muscular and mental 'holding on', but essentially, stationary pressure or connection at the appropriate angle and depth is what differentiates shiatsu from massage.

An exact description of how and why shiatsu works and how it is applied is presented in this book. In addition, I hope to convey that the quality and effectiveness of shiatsu is dependant upon the state of mind of the giver. For example, shiatsu demands an ability to patiently still and focus the mind in order to detect subtle changes within the receiver's vitality. Thereafter, it requires humility and skill to assist the natural healing process. It works more deeply if we understand that we cannot help restore true health effectively if we fail to acknowledge and respond to the person's particular energetic rhythm and distribution of Ki. The shiatsu practitioner learns to listen to those energies and assist their natural inclination towards balance and harmony. Shiatsu is therefore about skilfully nurturing the body/mind's potential for regaining vitality.

The required level of 'mindfulness' will naturally equip the giver with a greater ability to empathize with the receiver. This is because during the actual giving of shiatsu, the giver's mind is not in the future predicting the outcome of the session, or in the past trying to figure out why the receiver is as they are. The mind of the shiatsu therapist is trained to be in the 'here and now', which is the only time and space where we can hope to perceive 'reality'. What the receiver is experiencing during the shiatsu session is happening only in the present, as the sum total of all preceding factors bringing them to this moment. Therefore, shiatsu brings both the giver and receiver to the same point in time, known as '*now*'. To be 'aware' at that point in time, and aware of that point in time is the only condition in which empathy can be experienced. We all experience empathy at certain times. Those are the times when our consciousness rests for longer in the present.

In shiatsu we aspire to keep our consciousness relating to the present for as much of the session as possible. Most methods of meditation and 'mindfulness' have the same purpose. In that sense, shiatsu is as much a practice for developing growth in awareness, as it is a physical therapy. It is not mechanically physical, but rather physically mindful.

This book describes what is covered in a short shiatsu course for beginners. It should give you an insight into how to develop the qualities of conscious touch as just described. It is not intended to bring you to the point of consummation of those abilities. To acquire all the ingredients necessary for such a feat will require a thorough in-depth training in shiatsu therapy lasting several years. Even then, such a course can only be expected to equip you with the theory, techniques and 'tools' of shiatsu rather than the perfection of ability. Only the sustained patient practice of shiatsu following a legitimate and thorough training will give you the necessary skill and humility to call yourself a professional shiatsu practitioner. However, for the relief of stress and minor ailments amongst family and friends via the inducement of a very deep level of relaxation, skills learned on a short course can be applied immediately and to good effect.

It can be said that what you learn during the early phases of any subject tends to become more easily ingrained than those things learned later on. Consequently, if you learn inaccuracies and poor form in the beginning, it is much more difficult to correct them later. The true purpose of this book is to supplement a good quality beginner's course or foundation course in its proven method of getting the beginner student on the right track in their development of accurate and effective shiatsu technique.

You certainly cannot learn shiatsu solely from a book. Detailed personal instruction and close supervision is required. Please use this book as a useful companion to a comprehensive foundation course, or as an inspiration to partake of such a course. Then keep this book as a constant reminder of basic shiatsu technique and principles, which will remain the same whatever level you end up taking your shiatsu to. If in months or years to come you look back through this book and find that what you are doing under the name of shiatsu contradicts or bears little relation to what is said within it, then that is the time to re-read this book carefully. That is not to say this book represents a dogma or the last word on shiatsu technique; but it does elucidate the factors that make shiatsu what it is. Feel free to develop new techniques or reinterpret the theory as you gain experience. Once you are truly skilled there are no limits to the possibilities of adding to shiatsu. Just be careful not to let go of the core. A solid snowball will grow as it rolls, but not if its original core melts.

# The origins of shiatsu

Shiatsu is a method of bodywork formulated in Japan in the 20th Century. It is a Japanese development of various older forms of Chinese bodywork that are still practised in China and elsewhere today. In common with acupuncture and Chinese herbal medicine, these Chinese bodywork methods are all based on the principles of traditional Oriental medicine; which also originated in ancient China. The degree to which shiatsu incorporates traditional Oriental medicine varies according to the 'style' of shiatsu practised.

In the first half of the 20th Century, Oriental medicine was generally discouraged throughout Japan in favour of Western medicine, and many leading anma and shiatsu exponents abandoned their heritage of Oriental medicine. However, some, along with many of their contemporaries in acupuncture, worked towards re-establishing Oriental medicine in Japan. Although the predominant style of shiatsu in Japan is still mostly Western medicine based, the latter third of the 20th Century has seen a complete reintegration of traditional Oriental medicine into many styles of shiatsu; particularly those now practised in the West.

Whichever style of shiatsu is practised, they all share many fundamental principles of how to apply pressure and stretch. All styles have some techniques influenced by modern Western osteopathic or chiropractic methods; particularly in regard to muscle lengthening and mobilizing joints.

Today, shiatsu continues to grow and develop as its roots in Oriental medicine are explored ever more deeply. Modern practitioners and teachers are developing more methods of developing sensitivity to Ki and of 'reading' the body, as well as innovative ways to apply effective technique based on the theories of Oriental medicine.

# How to use this book

The chapters in this book reiterate most of the information you would be presented with on a comprehensive shiatsu beginner's course. Thus, they will remind you how to prepare yourself physically and mentally, apply technique correctly, and help you understand and remember the reason why we do shiatsu the way we do; and why it has the effect it has. Each chapter is profusely illustrated to give you as great a visual reminder as is possible within a book.

If you skim through this book, you will gain a clear visual impression of efficiently performed shiatsu techniques. If you take your time and read the chapters studiously, you will have a good understanding of the shiatsu principles required to give de-stressing shiatsu to your family or friends. Basic concepts of theory and practice are presented within the first few chapters, but for those of you who want to glean a little more in-depth shiatsu theory, this information is located towards the end of the book.

## Beyond the beginner's level

Once you have completed a comprehensive beginner's course in shiatsu, based on the same or similar techniques to those outlined in this book, you will be equipped with all the tools necessary to give a general full body shiatsu; thus helping to rebalance the strength and flow of the person's Ki, as well as improve the circulation of their blood and body fluids. If you then decide to study to full practitioner level, you will gain a deeper understanding of shiatsu practice and theory, along with a greater degree of sensitivity to Ki imbalances through the development of diagnostic skills. A practitioner course will teach you a wide range of practical techniques, including ways to affect all the Ki channels throughout the body, therapeutic stretching, how to develop your own style and how to formulate treatments for a variety of health problems. You will also receive a thorough grounding in the theories of Oriental medicine and in Western anatomy, physiology and pathology. Before receiving a diploma you will also carry out some form of clinical work and learn how to manage a shiatsu practice.

While the curriculum for a diploma course may look very complex, the subject matter is actually very logical and builds naturally upon the basics of shiatsu. It is simple to master provided you can give the necessary time to build up your touch sensitivity and read around the subject. The rewards are great, in that you will have a skill that will genuinely help others as well as yourself.

# CHAPTER 1

# How Shiatsu Works

This book deals primarily with the practical aspects of effective shiatsu technique. However, to get you into the swing of things, I have, in this chapter, briefly described those key concepts of theory which will enable you to grasp why shiatsu works.

## The Concept of Ki and Channels (Meridians)

Shiatsu works by helping to harmonize the energy and vitality of the body and mind. We know that when we eat we acquire energy, and if we eat healthily we expect to have more vitality. We also know that our quality of breathing is directly related to our energy levels. But what is it that animates us so that we are able to breathe and eat, move around and think? Something other than food and air exists within all living things, causing them to be 'alive'. Also, once 'life' has truly left the body, it has never, as far as we know, been successfully put back.

Western traditions view our 'life force' as an esoteric phenomenon, generally accepted by us as a gift from greater powers. As such, westerners have not tried to understand it to the extent their oriental counterparts have. The oriental traditions see our 'aliveness' and therefore our energy and vitality as much more to do with our interaction with surrounding nature and the universe. Daoist philosophy, from which the bulk of Far Eastern medicine bases itself, is basically a way of describing and understanding how our environment and ourselves function together. It is to do with understanding how all things are ultimately striving to maintain balance and harmony; and the observation that absolute balance and harmony cannot exist, due to constant opposing forces at work throughout nature.

Western thought has a rich fund of detailed information pertaining to how we are affected by cosmological cycles: astrology being the obvious example. However, it seems that it is the oriental philosophies that most clearly map out how nature and our body/mind is animated and functions (see Chapter 8). Here, we can simply say that the difference between that which is alive and that which is not alive is the presence or absence of 'aliveness'. This 'aliveness' is called Ki in Japanese, Qi or Ch'i in Chinese and Prana in Sanskrit (an ancient language of the Indian sub-continent). As this book is about shiatsu, we will call it Ki.

While we are alive, Ki or 'aliveness' permeates every part of our body, keeping each cell and every bodily function alive. Although cells are dying throughout our body, they are being constantly replaced. Cell replacement reduces as we get older, until not enough of the essential ones necessary for correct organic functioning are replaced. At that time we malfunction and die. The more Ki that reaches the cells, the less prone to decay they will be; so that an abundant supply of Ki to a cell means a healthier cell. However, it is not simply a question of quantity, but also of movement. All living things exhibit more activity than dead versions of the same. Ki is flowing smoothly and abundantly in a cycle within healthy vibrant creatures. Unhealthy creatures are not vibrant, because their Ki is not flowing smoothly.

It may be that Ki is not present in sufficient quantity to generate sufficient momentum to allow for a smooth flow, resulting in areas being starved of vitality while other areas stagnate and accumulate waste products; rather like insufficient water failing to flush debris from a pipe. Alternatively, it may be that too much Ki is accumulating in a particular area or function of the body, causing stagnation or hyper-activity there; rather like too many cars on a constricted road, resulting in no cars moving, causing potential or actual irritation and aggression (road rage in traffic jams?). So, to remain healthy or to regain health, Ki must be restored if it is deficient, unblocked if it is stuck and calmed if it is irritated. It must be kept moving.

Imbalances of Ki have many causes, including the effect of emotional disturbance, shock, mental attitude, abnormal environmental factors such as excessive heat or cold, extreme assault from virulent organisms, poisons, poor diet, incorrect use of the body (creating stress on the posture and organs), accidents and so on. A professional shiatsu practitioner will strive to identify the cause and the exact effect of that cause upon the person seeking treatment. However, the net result will be that the practitioner will apply shiatsu to enhance Ki where needed, disperse and/or calm the Ki where it is blocked or 'irritated', and make sure it circulates smoothly. Based on the understanding of what caused the imbalance, the practitioner will usually give some advice as to how to avoid those situations or factors that exacerbate the problem. All successful healing arts do this. Shiatsu, and other oriental body therapies achieve it by addressing the Ki directly.

To understand the essence of shiatsu, you should know that Ki is flowing everywhere throughout the living body, but aggregates into *channels* of more concentrated Ki flow. Here is an analogy: If the sea is full of water, then some areas of the sea will have stronger currents, resulting from the dynamic movement and interaction of the sea and the planet as a whole. Many of these currents can be charted (such as the gulf stream). Likewise, within a human or animal body, the general dynamic of being alive will result in Ki aggregating along chartable courses. Over the millenia, the Chinese have mapped out these channels, often called *meridians*, and through centuries of observation, noticed what happens when a channel does not flow in the way it should. Consequently, they devised ways of restoring the correct 'attitude' of the channels and the Ki within them. The Chinese ancestry to Japanese shiatsu was one such method. Modern shiatsu is still based on these core principles.

These channels or 'meridians' run like rivers all over the surface of the body, continuing like subterranean rivers deep into the interior of the body, directing Ki into and from all the internal organs. Where one channel begins and ends, it continues into another channel, so that you have a continuous circuit. Sometimes a channel will also connect with one or more other channels elsewhere along its course. From the *main* or *primary* channels, stream-like branches divide off at intervals, which themselves sub-divide into more streams to supply Ki to all the bodily structures, such as muscles, fascia, bone and so on. The channel system is like a vast matrix supplying Ki to, and allowing intercommunication of Ki between, all areas and functions of the body. This is not dissimilar to the ever dividing and spreading profile of our nervous system and circulatory systems.

In shiatsu, as in the other branches of Oriental medicine, the internal organs are related to a wide range of functions of both the body and the mind. As such, if you affect the Ki channel of the receiver of shiatsu in some way, there will, at some level, be an effect upon their bodily functions, emotions and psychological disposition. A more comprehensive description of these functions is given on pages 141–155. An outline of the 14 primary channels is given on pages 158–185. This is the essence of a shiatsu session: *to help the person's Ki re-establish strength and a more harmonious free flowing state through the skilled and aware application of physical contact to the body surface, thus bringing all aspects of the body/mind into greater harmony.*

## Tsubos (Pressure Points)

At specific locations along the Ki channels (hereafter referred to as channels), there are 'gateways' or 'cavities' where Ki can open to the surface. These gateways are known as *tsubos* and are essentially points where Ki can:

A. Access the channel from outside the body;
B. Leave the channel to connect with the outside world; or
C. Represent distortions in the channel flow, so that when 'activated' (by pressure for example) can affect the channel, and therefore affect some aspect of body/mind function.

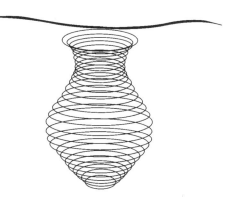

*A representation of the tsubo vortex.*

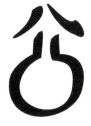

*The Japanese character for tsubo.*

A tsubo is a vortex of Ki that, if you could see it, would look like a vase shaped swirl of energy with a mouth leading into a narrower neck, widening into a broader belly; as shown below. Also shown below is the Japanese written character for tsubo, which illustrates this concept perfectly.

Each of the primary channels has a number of *fixed* tsubos. Generations of documented observation has resulted in each tsubo being given a name, number and recognized action on the body and mind when stimulated.

In addition to the fixed tsubos, there are *transient* tsubos which come and go along the channels between the fixed tsubos. They arise where and when they do because there is either a lack of Ki or an excessive build up of Ki at that location and at that point in time along the channel. Where the Ki is lacking, the tsubo will feel lifeless and empty, lacking vitality and elasticity. It may be stiff and lifeless or flaccid and lifeless. Sometimes it may be flaccid and lifeless on the surface and stiff and lifeless deeper down. Where the Ki is blocked and consequently overcrowded, there will be a feeling of fullness, tightness and constriction at that location, often accompanied by pain when touched there. Sometimes the full areas will feel warm whereas the deficient areas will feel cold.

Very occasionally, the shiatsu practitioner will feel active resistance on contacting a tsubo, even if the tsubo is deficient in Ki, thus making it difficult to discern whether it is full or empty. This is because surrounding Ki will rush to protect the empty 'vulnerable' tsubo. This only happens when the tsubo is approached too quickly or too forcefully; which should not happen if your Shiatsu is applied correctly. To understand this concept more fully, see pages 15–17, 'Metaphors to Explain Kyo/Jitsu').

Shiatsu is a method of bodywork that largely focuses on methods to re-balance the activity of Ki in and around the tsubos.

## Ki Imbalance

To be alive is to have sufficient Ki to enable our body/mind to react in some way. To be dead is to have insufficient Ki to react at all. The way Ki manifests in our actions and reactions depends upon what external factors are bearing down upon us, what our immediate needs are and how emotionally and physically at ease we are within ourselves. So, if we possess sufficient Ki and are completely satisfied, our Ki will be evenly distributed throughout our body, smoothly transported through our network of Ki channels, giving us the appearance of being at rest. On the other hand, as soon as a need arises, such as hunger, we are no longer in a state of complete satisfaction. Hunger means we want food. As such, our Ki will aggregate into specific areas and functions of our body/mind (and therefore into specific Ki channels and tsubos) to enable us to get food. Therefore, if you are sat down without hunger, you might as well stay sat down. But if you are really hungry, your Ki will move into all the muscles that enable you to get up and reach the food. If the food is just an arms length away, very little Ki will need to be redistributed for you to eat. However, if you have to run after, catch, kill, prepare, guard and eat your food, then a lot more Ki will need to be reorganized within you. Once the hunger has been satisfied, your Ki distribution can return to its balanced state.

From this analogy, we can see that any activity we engage in results from a desire or need to fulfil ourselves. Getting food is an obvious example. But even the activity of drawing a picture results from a desire to draw it. That desire would not exist if we were totally fulfilled and satiated. We might draw the picture out of the emptiness of boredom, or the belief that the world must have this picture. Whatever the specific motivation is for drawing the picture, the underlying thought is that we believe the picture should come into existence. Until the picture is completed to our satisfaction, we will invest a great deal of Ki into the functions that enable us to draw it. Once the picture is drawn, our Ki will return to balance.

So, all activity and therefore all movement of Ki within a living being, results from need. The fluctuation from need to fulfilment continues as long as life continues. It is perfectly normal, but it explains why Ki actually moves more into certain channels and tsubos at any given time. As long as the Ki does return to normal, we remain healthy. However, if it remains stuck and does not rebalance itself, the seeds of ill health are born. It can remain stuck because our intellect and our relationship to our environment is so complex that we do not clearly recognize what our needs are and often fail to see when they are fulfilled. The simpler the intellect of a life form, the more linear is the process of fulfilling basic needs. For a slug, life revolves around the emptiness of hunger that then leads to the act of eating; and the instinct to procreate with the act of sexual intercourse. A spider is much the same, but seems to have a greater instinct or 'desire' for survival, judging from the way they scurry away when you approach them. But for us humans, although we have the same basic instincts and needs as other animals, our intelligence both clarifies and confuses our reason for living. Do you eat only when you are hungry? Do you sometimes eat to satisfy a desire, only to find that it did not satisfy that desire? .. as if you even knew what that desire was! Why do some people wreck themselves trying to accumulate more food or money than they need? Why can't that colleague accept who they are and stop trying to change into who or what they are not?

The answers to such questions may be found through reflection, philosophy and psychology. What concerns the shiatsu practitioner is what the effect of all this has on the distribution of Ki within the receiver's body, and what he or she can do to help rebalance the Ki.

## Kyo-Jitsu

In shiatsu terminology, fullness or excess of Ki causing blockage or hyper-activity in a channel or tsubo is referred to as *jitsu*, whereas deficiency or emptiness of Ki resulting in hypo-activity or relative 'lifelessness' in a channel is known as *kyo*. To further understand kyo, consider that every part of a living body seeks to be nourished by Ki and blood, so if insufficient Ki reaches any part, then that part exhibits a 'need' for more Ki. Furthermore, a need (kyo) will eventually create a reaction (jitsu) somewhere, in an attempt to compensate for, or to meet that need. Kyo is therefore the underlying cause for jitsu. To reiterate the analogy of hunger, if the food supply is ample, there is no need to urgently rush around to fill the food cabinets (which is analogous to the channel in relative balance). However, if the food runs out and we start to go hungry, we begin to focus a lot of energy and resources into procuring more food (the 'needy' kyo channel area is causing heightened activity or 'jitsu' elsewhere). When some family members start to grow dangerously weak from hunger, those who can will go to extreme lengths to get food (greater kyo leads to more intense jitsu elsewhere). In a way, we are like a huge fabric or matrix that wants to be evenly spread. So when an imbalance in one area causes distortion in other areas, a lot of energy is used in an attempt to restore equilibrium.

The Ki matrix of the body/mind, which is made up of our Ki channels, instinctively strives for balance. It wants smooth flow of Ki and a trouble free existence. But our minds, our activities and environmental influences sometimes work against that. Yet our Ki matrix still strives for harmony within itself. It actually takes a lot of effort or adverse circumstance to overcome the harmony of the body. However, when the balance is lost, we get ill. Even then, the illness itself is an attempt to restore harmony. But sometimes the body/mind just does not have the final resources or resolve to get well without some outside help. Hence, we have healing systems of various sorts, including shiatsu, which helps restore health or prevent ill health by basically helping to keep the Ki flowing smoothly throughout the channels, by using techniques to meet the needs of the kyo and if necessary, disperse or calm down the jitsu.

So, any given channel will exhibit some areas that are more kyo areas and others that are more jitsu. In addition, you can expect any channel when viewed overall, to err towards more kyo or more jitsu in relation to other channels. The whole 'matrix' is constantly fluctuating. A shiatsu therapist will find the most kyo channel and the most jitsu channel and focus their work on these two. By moving some of the Ki from the Jitsu channel to the Kyo channel, they will enhance the Ki within the kyo channel, therefore fulfilling its need for Ki.

The jitsu areas are easier to find because they feel 'active' and react locally to pressure. Jitsu areas sometimes protrude from the surface. Kyo areas are more difficult to locate because they exhibit little or no reaction to touch, and do not generally manifest an obvious presence on the surface, although the trained eye and trained touch can often see or feel kyo as a depression or 'sinking' into the surface. However, that is still more difficult than seeing that which protrudes or feeling that which reacts. The following chart gives some comparisons of kyo and jitsu.

### Some Comparisons of Kyo and Jitsu

| *Kyo* | *Jitsu* |
| --- | --- |
| A 'need' which requires the Ki to be supported and strengthened. | A bodily reaction representing its natural attempt to restore harmonious Ki flow. |
| Underlying cause. | Manifests as symptoms. |
| Empty – requires filling. | Full – requires emptying / dispersing. |
| 'Stagnation' in the channel due to the lack of Ki being unable to sustain enough momentum for Ki circulation. | 'Stagnation' in the channel due to too much Ki occupying a confined area (like a traffic jam). |
| Underactive, leading to flaccidity or stiffness. | Hyperactive, leading to congestion, blockage and impenetrability. |
| Below surface. | Protruding from surface. |
| Less obvious. | More obvious. |
| Slower to respond. | Immediate response. |
| Requires deep, sustained connection. | Requires moving/active technique or to be left alone. |
| Its tonification affects the whole person. | Its dispersal affects localized body areas. |

Certain external factors such as a cold wind blowing down your neck might cause the Ki in some of the channels running through that area to block or react in some way. This reaction is a response to the external influence, namely, the wind; rather than some kyo elsewhere in the body. However, if out of three people exposed to the same situation, only one gets a stiff neck from Ki blockage, what is it about that person which is different from the other two? The answer is: that person had some underlying weakness compared to the other two people, which means his resistance to wind was lower. So ultimately, if not immediately or obviously, jitsu always manifests out of a response to kyo.

Balancing kyo and jitsu distortions in the channels and tsubos constitutes the bulk of shiatsu technique application, although there are other facets to its practice. At the beginners level it is not necessary to worry too much about developing highly skilled methods for recognizing and dealing with kyo and jitsu. That can all come with further training. At this level you can begin by simply recognizing where your touch is not welcome and avoiding those areas, and recognizing where your touch is appreciated or 'wanted', and applying sustained contact to those 'appreciative' areas. You can ask the receiver to tell you whether they want you to continue adding pressure to an area or whether they want you to move away from that area. They will definitely tell you if you give them permission, because the jitsu areas will hurt them if pressure is applied. So when they say stop, you stop and move on. After some practice, you will begin to recognize the signs well before they have to tell you to quit the technique; thus your sensitivity will grow.

**Metaphors to Explain Kyo-Jitsu**

You can equate your approach to a Kyo or Jitsu tsubo with the way you might approach a herd of deer grazing in a meadow. In a small clearing in the woods to one side of the meadow, two stags are locked in conflict over who is to be the dominant male of the herd. This situation arises during the mating season, but on this occasion the stag conflict is heightened by the fact that a fawn has been badly injured. The stag's innate desire to become the dominant male sire is exacerbated by an instinct to be the chief herd protector.

*Tonifying blocked/full jitsu (doomed to failure).*

Imagine these deer are relatively tame, so you could get close to them if you approached them with care. You want to come close to the stags to study their aggressive behaviour, but that would not be a good idea because the stags are confined within the clearing in the woods and very much preoccupied with their struggle. There is already too much tense energy around and your presence would add to it. If you persist in trying to get between them, the aggression of both stags will increase and they will turn on you. They do not want you around any more than a jitsu tsubo would want your thumb trying to get into it. The sensible thing is to leave the stags alone for now.

*Dispersing blocked/full jitsu (without tonifying kyo).*

If you collected some friends together and rushed at the stags, making as much noise and commotion as possible, they would scatter, at which point you and your friends leave the scene. For a while, the concentrated activity in that corner of the woods has been forcibly removed. However, when the coast is clear the stags return. If you and your friends rushed them again, the stags may not scatter so easily a second time, being more accustomed to your presence. This is akin to dispersing jitsu by applying active technique directly to it, but without directing it to a kyo area. The Ki scatters randomly, only to return to the same place later on with more tenacity and stubbornness.

*Calming hyperactive jitsu.*

Standing on the edge of the scene is a young stag that is becoming excited. Though he is rather slight in build and but a shadow of the hefty mature stags, he is frenetically rushing around, filling his space with jittery energy. You approach him and offer him a handful of grass, which he finds quite appealing. You then radiate a very calm demeanour, holding your calming hand to his back. The young stag eventually settles down to graze calmly, because deep down he knows that he is not sufficiently mature to engage in mating rituals. This is like placing a calming hand on the type of jitsu that does not represent excess quantity of Ki, but rather, excess activity within a limited quantity of Ki.

*Tonifying mild rather than chronic kyo, that is, resistance at the surface (simultaneously dispersing jitsu via 'two-hand connection').*

The wounded fawn's mother and a few other close relatives are staying close to the fawn to protect it. You are there with a first aid kit, intending to help the fawn. But how are those protecting the fawn to know you want to help? To them, you pose a threat, but they also have a sixth sense suggesting that you might in fact be trying to help. They are confused, so you approach very slowly, stopping whenever there is a hint of panic. You give enough space and time for them to become accustomed to the idea of your offer to help. At no stage must you assume acceptance and rush in to finish the job. The same can apply to a kyo tsubo. Sometimes you detect a 'need' for more Ki, but when you try to apply perpendicular pressure, surrounding Ki aggregates at the neck of the tsubo, preventing further entry.

Once you reach the fawn and you are clearly helping it rather than harming it, its protectors back off a little and the whole scene becomes more relaxed. You administer some medicine that gives the fawn some vitality (some Ki) and the fawn struggles to its feet.

If you have a colleague called 'support hand' who can tell the stag that it is worthwhile helping the herd to aid and protect the recovering fawn, that can be viewed as an analogy for the Ki in the jitsu tsubo being alerted to, and guided towards, the kyo tsubo.

*Comparative response of blocked, hyperactive or empty 'needy' tsubo to stationary perpendicular pressure.*

The longer you stay motionless at the mouth of the kyo tsubo, the more the resistance dissipates, allowing you further entry as long as you do not push. Conversely, the longer you linger at the mouth of the full jitsu tsubo, the more intolerant the Ki becomes and resistance actually increases. The only way to deal with the jitsu that is more frenetic than full is to use a palm rather than a thumb; to be calm and allow that calmness to subdue the jitsu activity. This is very similar in attitude to dealing with the protected kyo tsubo, except you would not try to enter the tsubo to add Ki.

*Tonifying more chronic, but not the most chronic, kyo: that is, flaccid kyo.*

Another scenario could be this: the fawn has been injured for a long time, is completely unconscious and inert. The herd have left it for dead and are grazing several hundred metres away. However, the mother remains on the edge of the herd, keeping the fawn in sight.

You can approach the fawn with no resistance. When you reach the fawn, you patiently administer some healing factor (Ki). After a while, the fawn stirs. This is noticed by the mother, who comes over to the fawn, along with others of the herd. You leave and allow the herd to support the revived fawn.

*Tonifying very chronic kyo: that is, stiff kyo.*

Yet another scenario: the fawn is dead and the herd is on the horizon. Even the mother deer has given up hope and forgotten about the fawn. You approach the fawn to see how it is. There is no resistance to your approach, but what you find when you reach the fawn is a stiff, inert carcass, analogous to a stiff, inert kyo tsubo.

When something is dead, the Ki, blood and body fluids no longer circulate to moisten, activate and nourish the body. When the creature has been dead for a while, the prolonged absence of Ki, blood and fluid function will result in a general drying and stiffening of the tissues. Likewise, kyo in part of a living body reflects the relative lack of life (Ki) in that part of the body. If the Ki is very deficient for a long time, blood and fluid circulation to that area will be drastically reduced, causing a drying out and atrophy of the tissues. The chronic kyo area will be virtually a 'dead' part of the body; a part that the owner will have very little awareness of, unless it is so dead that the tissues exhibit pathological problems (an extreme example would be gangrene).

No matter how much healing agent you give the fawn, it is dead and that is that. No matter how long you try to tonify that completely stiff, dead kyo, it will not respond. So what can you do? It makes more sense if, rather than concentrating on the dead fawn itself, you think of the dead fawn in terms of the space it is occupying being a dead space. All around, active creatures are bringing their living space alive. Because you persist in standing over the carcass, you mark the spot and eventually attract the attention of various predators, carrion feeders and other opportunists. In due course, the predators will come closer, and when you move off, they will eat the carcass, effectively causing renewed activity in that space; thereby bringing 'life' to that space.

Translated into the chronic stiff kyo situation, this means that if you hold patient, sustained perpendicular pressure on that lifeless tsubo, nothing whatsoever will happen. However, if you leave it and tonify and disperse more interactive parts of the body, you might well find that when you return, either during this treatment or within a later treatment, some activity has begun to manifest in that formerly stiff kyo tsubo.

## The Effect of Shiatsu on the Autonomic Nervous System (ANS)

Taken in its entirety, shiatsu therapy draws upon an extensive theoretical base and range of practical approaches, and can offer an almost endless selection of techniques. However, a correctly applied shiatsu session consisting of basic techniques only, without working specifically on the channels and without using the tools of diagnosis and Oriental medicine theory, will still have a tremendously positive effect upon the receiver. It is this level of basic shiatsu application that this book sets out to describe. In a nutshell, shiatsu at any level, is incredibly relaxing, revitalizing and it strengthens our immune system. This is because it invokes the para-sympathetic response of the autonomic nervous system, which in simple terms means a deep relaxation response.

For our purposes here, there is no need for an exhaustive discussion of the physiology of the autonomic nervous system; it is sufficient to understand that we have physiological and psychological responses to threat, which are more or less opposite to our reaction to safe and supportive situations.

When we perceive ourselves to be under threat, we become very alert so that we can rapidly assess the gravity and detail of the situation, thereby giving ourselves the optimum chance to counteract or escape from that which threatens us. Depending on the level of threat, we may be required to defend ourselves, either by fighting it out or by running away. Under threat, our bodies will automatically send more adrenaline into the blood and more blood to the muscles, ensuring their optimum performance. Our breathing rhythm will accelerate to ensure enough oxygen gets to our muscles and brain, and our senses of hearing, seeing and smelling will become more acute. We become ready for action. On the other hand, when we feel safe and not under pressure, we tend to let go and relax. Our breathing slows down and our eyes and ears become less sharply focused.

If you touch someone in the correct way, at the appropriate time and with the right attitude, the touch will soothe and support them. No doubt you have experienced at least a hand on your shoulder from the right person at the right time when you were upset. It helped, did it not? Conversely, that shove from someone who saw you as nothing more than an object in their way made you feel irritated, and your muscles tensed up.

*The Japanese character for human.*

So, if you push someone, you can expect him or her to tense up and take up a closed defensive posture, or even an aggressive stance towards you. If you offer a supportive contact, such as catching someone as they trip over, their attitude to you is likely to be positive and this will be reflected in a lessening of their bodily tensions when interacting with you. Try leaning against a good friend when you appear to be tired; they will instinctively support you. Then push them and see what happens! It is interesting that the Japanese written character for human suggests that to be leaned on rather than to be pushed is fundamental to human co-operation. It implies that benevolent human contact makes both us and those we come into contact with, more human.

Shiatsu technique emphasizes this leaning, 'humanizing' principle. You always lean rather than push to apply pressure. In other words, pressure is applied using your body weight rather than with muscular strength. Exactly how you do this is covered in Chapter 3.

# CHAPTER 2

# Preparing to Give Shiatsu

This chapter looks at how to set the scene for a successful shiatsu session, which is as relevant to basic shiatsu as it is to professional shiatsu therapy. It covers how to prepare your body, how to prepare your mind, and how to prepare your working environment.

In addition to being sufficiently mobile on the ground, the giver of shiatsu needs to work on his or her own health in as many ways as possible. You will not give such a good shiatsu if you do not feel well. Also those with less vitality (less Ki) will tend to gravitate towards those with more vitality, because one tends to seek in others what one lacks in oneself. So in order to attract people to practice shiatsu on, you should try to be at least as healthy as they are. Ki, vitality or whatever you want to call it, tends to flow from the one with the greater supply to the one with the lesser supply. Therefore, you are not going to help the receiver of your shiatsu if your Ki is depleted in comparison to them. In fact, you could drain them of their vitality and cause them to feel a lot worse. As a giver of hands on bodywork, you should strive to keep your Ki clear and strong.

Most shiatsu practitioners practice some form of meditation, yoga, taiji quan or qigong; all of which, if done correctly and with sufficient diligence, will improve one's Ki.

## How to Prepare Your Body: the Makko-ho Positions

Shiatsu is normally given at floor level, rather than on a couch or table. For this reason it requires the giver to be able to move around with ease on the floor. Therefore, of particular relevance are exercises that help to keep your legs, hips, pelvis and spine supple. A system of exercises known as the *Makko-ho positions*, which is practised widely by shiatsu practitioners and students, fulfils this aim. In addition, the Makko-ho positions open each pair of channels, enabling you to monitor whether the Ki in any particular channel is blocked or weak. Both blocked and weak Ki will tend to manifest as stiffness during the exercise, although weakness of Ki can sometimes show as hyper-mobility accompanied by a sense of instability in those joints most closely associated with the movement. In other words, where a channel is more jitsu, the exercise will be difficult due to stiffness. For a channel that is more kyo, the exercise may feel stiff, or it may feel easy, but a bit wobbly. Until you know exactly where the channels are, this nuance will not be so relevant. Pages 158–185 present diagrams of the channel locations, for those of you who wish to explore this aspect. However, the positions are effective whether you are familiar with channel location or not.

When doing the Makko-ho positions, try to remain relaxed throughout, except where stated otherwise; as in some exercises where I have indicated a part of the body which you should contract while relaxing the rest of your body. The following checklist applies to each position:

- Breathe in.
- Move into the position as you breathe out.
- Check that everything is relaxed.
- Remain in the position and breathe in again.
- Exhale and try to let go a little more.
- See if you can passively allow yourself to relax a little further into the position.
- Never bounce or push yourself into the position; go very slowly and stop where it still feels comfortable.
- Do three or four long and slow exhalations while 'dwelling' in each position.
- Carry out the exercises in the order given, because the effect of each position is designed to be enhanced by the previous one and to enhance the following one.

Don't worry if you fail to get very far into any position; it is the *intention without expectation* that counts here. All exercises from the sitting position tend to be easier if the buttocks are raised on a stiff cushion or block of 2–4 inches (5–10 cm) in depth.

You can do these exercises any time of day, but you will be stiffer in the morning than in the evening, so remember to take that into account.

The effects of these exercises are enhanced if you consider the emotional or psychological function of the channels affected, from the perspective of Oriental medicine (as indicated in italic). However, they will still be effective if you choose to ignore that aspect.

To minimize the risk of injury for readers who are not used to doing exercises of this nature, I have made some minor amendments to some of the original Makko-ho positions, based on modern research into body mechanics.

## Lung/Large Intestine

This exercise facilitates a more efficient *intake of Ki* by opening the Lung channel and enhances the ability to *let go* (both physically and emotionally) by activating the Large Intestine channel. Go into the position very slowly and come up equally slowly.

Note: Keep your knees bent if you have slight problems with your back, and avoid bending forward at all if you have severe back problems or very low blood pressure.

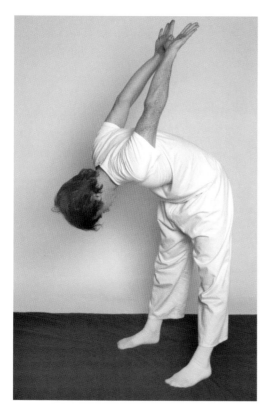
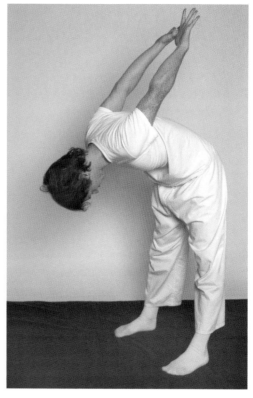

*Stand with your feet hip-width apart and link your thumbs behind your back. Lean forward, dropping your head.*

*Stretch your hands away from your shoulder blades rather than over and beyond your head. Keep your knees slightly bent unless you are used to similar exercises such as forward-stretching yoga postures.*

## Stomach/Spleen

These channels relate to our *desire to grasp food*. That could be why these channels are on the front of the body, because when you're really hungry, you tend to go forwards rather than backwards to get food!

Do not do this if you have a lower back problem or inflamed knees, and go down further than shown in the picture only if you have total confidence in your own flexibility. Below are two variations that largely eliminate potential strain on your lower back and knees.

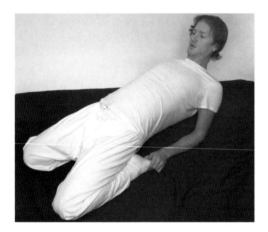

*Kneel down with your feet tucked back and with your buttocks on the floor or on a cushion. Rest back on your elbows. Keep your buttocks as tightly clenched as possible to counteract potential strain on your lower back. Puff out your chest and keep your chin tucked in. Go back further only if you are confident in your own flexibility. Go down very slowly and come up equally slowly.*

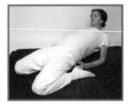 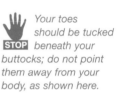

*Your toes should be tucked beneath your buttocks; do not point them away from your body, as shown here.*

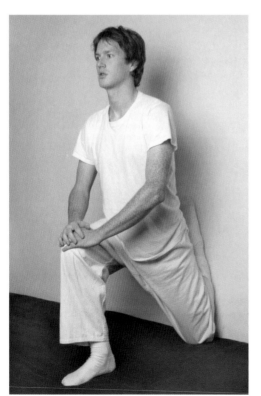

*To eliminate potential strain on lower back and knees, kneel with your left knee against the wall, resting your buttocks against your heel. Your right leg should be bent at a right angle, foot on the floor. Contract your buttocks and bring your lower back towards the wall as far as is reasonably achievable. Lift your arms overhead if you want maximum stretch. Repeat on the other leg.*

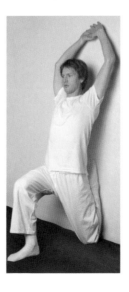

### Heart/Small Intestine

The Heart relates to our *raw awareness* or *consciousness*, whereas the Small Intestine enables us to *assimilate mental concepts* and *information*, as well as assimilate food. This exercise involves folding yourself around your centre, which will naturally make you feel more *calm and centred*. It brings your awareness to areas on the inner surface of your body that relate to the Heart, and simultaneously opens the Small Intestine channel.

*Clasp your feet in front of you as close to your groin as you can, with your knees spread apart. Curl forwards in a relaxed way, tuning into the feeling of 'inward attention'. Your elbows should be outside and in front of your shins.*

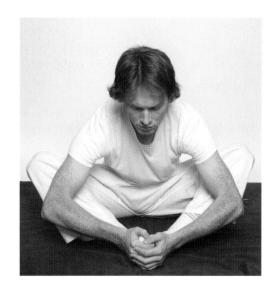

### Bladder/Kidney

This exercise opens and frees the back of the torso and legs, giving those areas sufficient Ki to ensure you can stand up straight and *stand your ground, and go forward in life with confidence*. Do not pull on your feet or ankles. Go down very slowly and come up equally slowly. NEVER FORCE THIS POSITION.

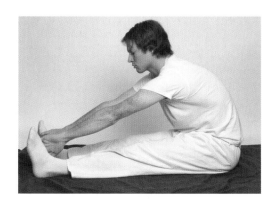

*Sitting with your legs straight out in front of you, bend forward from your hips and place your hands, palms turned out, between your feet, with your little fingers uppermost. Aim your navel towards your thighs, not your head towards your feet.*

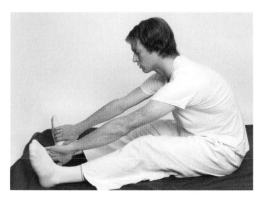

*If you are particularly stiff in the hamstrings or have lower back problems, bend your knees a little and focus on any sensations you feel in the back of your legs. This will help activate the Bladder and Kidney channels. If you legs can almost straighten, it may help to have your buttocks raised 2–4 inches (5–10 cm) on a firm cushion or block. If you cannot reach your feet even with your knees slightly bent, hold your ankles.*

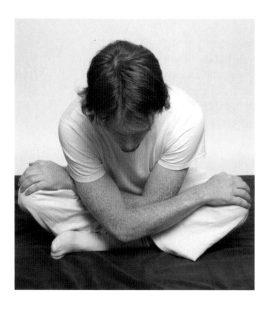

### Heart Protector/Triple Heater

The Heart Protector (also referred to as Pericardium) protects the Heart both physically and emotionally (helping you avoid the devastation of a 'broken heart'!). The Triple Heater, also referred to as Sanjiao, at one level, gives us a sense of *protection* against more general outside influences. Therefore, this enclosed Makko-ho position gives us a sense of our exposed outer shell (where the Triple Heater channel lies) protecting our soft inner Heart Protector channel. This position therefore gives us a general feeling of *protection and security*.

*Sit cross-legged and cross your arms the opposite way. Exhale as you curl forwards. Reverse your arms and legs and repeat.*

### Gallbladder/Liver

The Gallbladder has much to do with our courage to make decisions, whereas the Liver gives the *quality of foresight* and the ability to make plans. Both channels are principally involved in keeping our Ki flowing smoothly. As such, opening these channels, which involves a stretch to the side of your torso, activates an enhanced decisiveness about *which direction to take* in your life and in your day-to-day activities.

The order these exercises are done is in accordance with the Chinese Channel Clock Cycle (see page 156). While you do not need to refer to this, remember to carry out the exercises in the order shown above.

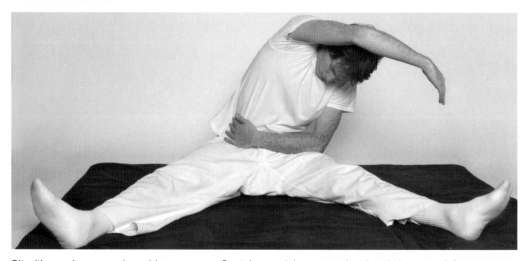

*Sit with your legs spread as wide as you can. Stretch your right arm overhead and place your left arm across your ribs. Lean down towards your left leg, constantly drawing your right shoulder back and your left shoulder forward, while opening your chest as much as you can so that your back remains as flat as possible. Do not crane your head forward or bend your knees. Do the exercise slowly, with awareness and without strain.*

## Qigong

Qigong is a word and concept from China. The broad and correct meaning of Qigong is: any training or study dealing with Qi (Ki) that takes a long time and great effort. In that sense, even shiatsu and acupuncture are forms of qigong. However, in modern use it has come to mean: practices, which encourage Qi development in the body, such as taiji qigong exercises. There are hundreds of qigong methods, each with many variations. Some emphasize stillness and internal visualization. Others emphasize slow movement, and some involve sudden spontaneous movements. All are designed to reap long term benefits resulting from long term practice, rather than as a quick way to feel good.

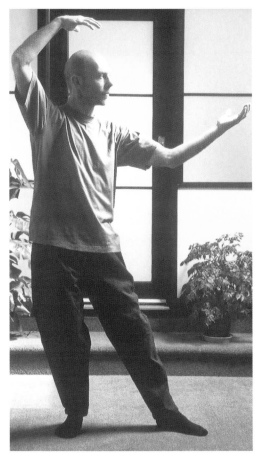

*A standing qigong exercise that is designed for calming the mind and grounding the body.*

# Do-In Exercises for the Hands and Feet

There is a system of Ki unblocking and Ki strengthening exercises known as Do-In (Japanese) or Dao-Yinn (Chinese). Do-In includes a wide range of stretching, acupressure, rubbing and percussion techniques that we can apply to ourselves. It is outside the scope of this book to describe Do-In in depth, but one simple aspect we can extract for our purposes here, is a preliminary Do-In method used to keep the joints of the hands and feet supple and free of blocked Ki. For the giver of shiatsu it is particularly helpful to keep Ki flowing smoothly throughout the hands and feet. This is because free flow of Ki in the feet helps to keep us grounded whereas smooth Ki flow through the hands ensures a better touch sensitivity and greater potential for the transmission of our healing touch. Traditionally performed at dawn, these exercises can be done at any time.

If you do these exercises when you get up in the morning, an excellent way of starting is to run your hands and feet under the cold tap. Your feet especially, will feel incredibly alive and warm afterwards, as blood and Ki rush into the feet. This feeling of aliveness will then quickly extend throughout your whole body. Keeping a box of pebbles under your bed to walk on immediately you get out of bed provides another good boost, providing a form of general reflexology 'tonic'.

You will be surprised at how much you can consciously influence the workings of your body if you can accept that Ki will go where your mind directs it. Therefore, if you clearly visualise stuck Ki exiting the wrist as fresh blood and Ki enters it, then that is what will happen. The more single-pointed your mental focus, the better this will work.

### Do-In exercise for the wrists

1.  *Apply a little traction to your wrist joint as you exhale, then release it (the arrow depicts traction). Now simply flap your wrist, keeping your wrist completely flaccid, holding an image in your mind of shaking out the debris of 'stuckness' and expelling Ki stagnation; rather like droplets of water spraying from a wet cloth from which you are trying to shake out excess water.*

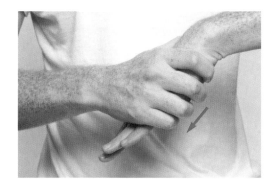

2.  *Hold both palms together in a prayer position with your hands held close to your chest and your elbows spread, thus extending your wrist joints. Move your hands down towards your waist until you feel the heels of your hands beginning to pull apart (the arrow shows the direction to descend the hands). Practice will result in your wrist flexibility improving, so that you can bring your hands progressively further down. Imagine all restriction to this movement melting away. You can then visualize clean oil working its way into all parts of the wrist joints.*

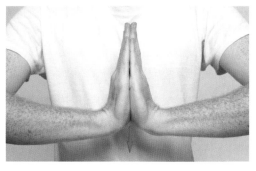

## Do-In for the fingers, ankles and toes

The following set of illustrations show a series of similar Do-In exercises for the fingers, ankles and toes. Follow the same principles and visualizations as the example just described for the wrist. Do not force any movement in any of these exercises.

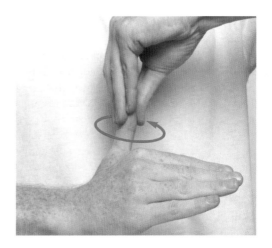

1. Take hold of your index finger and apply some traction to the finger as you rotate it. Rotate in both directions. Exhale as you apply the movement, visualizing increased blood flow and the expelling of waste products along with stagnant Ki. Repeat on all fingers in turn.

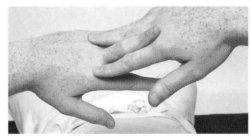

2. Make a 'fork' with your index and middle fingers and lever each finger of the other hand in turn, away from the palm, exhaling as you apply the movement. Imagine all restriction and stiffness melting away. Finish by flapping the hand and wrist.

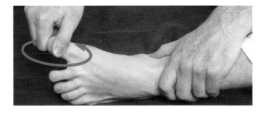

3. Take hold of your big toe and apply some traction to the toe as you rotate it. Rotate in both directions. Exhale as you apply the movement, visualizing increased blood flow and the expelling of waste products and stagnant Ki. Repeat on all your toes in turn.

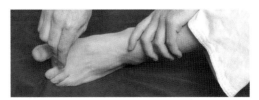

4. Gently lever each toe in turn towards the dorsum of the foot, exhaling as you apply the movement. Imagine all restriction and stiffness melting away. The third, fourth and fifth toes may even touch the dorsum of the foot within a few days of practice, but do not force them.

5. Beat the sole of your foot with your knuckles or fist for about 30 seconds. Be firm, but do not bruise yourself. Imagine you are beating the debris of Ki and blood stagnation out of the foot and ankle, thus dissolving all stiffness. When you stop, imagine you can feel all the pores in the sole of your foot 'breathing'. Finally, stand on one leg and vigorously shake your other foot in the air. As usual, imagine you are flushing out stagnation and poisons from your foot.

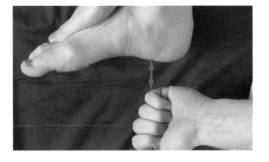

## Hatha Yoga Asanas

Every yoga asana (posture) will open and flush the Ki channels, assuming you do them correctly, even if they are not taught specifically with Ki channels in mind. (Energy pathways akin to Ki channels are known as *nadis* in yoga terminology). Yoga is now very popular, and if you decide to follow this route you should have no difficulty in finding classes locally.

## General Exercise and Ki

General exercise is great for maintaining and developing Ki; as long as it is non-destructive. By that I mean it is no point wrecking your joints in an attempt to build your Ki. The best exercises are those that encourage a full range of diverse movements that are not contrary to the way your musculo-skeletal system is designed to move. Walking, running (preferably over undulating terrain), swimming and so on are all great. The rule is:

- Moderate exercise smoothes and builds Ki.

- Excessive exercise exhausts and blocks Ki.

- No exercise at all tends to weaken your Ki.

Japanese Aikido masters often elect to manually tend their own land, as they consider the hard physical work involved helps keep their Ki strong.

If you exercise regularly, work enthusiastically and sleep sufficiently, the quality of your Ki will have a head start. If you then do some other deliberate Ki enhancing activities, your Ki will improve and develop quickly. It must not be forgotten that moving around the receiver as you give shiatsu involves a degree of exercise. If done well, giving shiatsu will benefit your Ki. Done badly, it will block your Ki and cause you discomfort, if not immediately, then later on.

## Nutrition

For every viewpoint on how to eat correctly, there is a completely opposite view claiming equal legitimacy. Should you eat only cooked food? All raw food? Less meat? More meat? Less grain? More grain? Nothing at all? Everything in sight? It can be very confusing. Once you know how and where to look and read between the lines, many apparent contradictions disappear. However, for most people it is a nightmare trying to figure it out.

To offer a few simple guidelines, I would suggest you avoid consistently eating junk food; but if you do so now and then, do not feel guilty about it. It is not what you eat on occasion that matters. What counts is what you eat regularly, as your staple diet. Even then, worrying about what you eat is likely to be far worse for you than actually eating it. Get some basic awareness of what is particularly not good and make a deal with yourself to generally avoid those things.

They say that to feel a little hungry after eating is good. This seems to be true, as long as it doesn't cause you to dwell upon that bit of food you did not have. If you really chew your food well, you will naturally avoid gorging yourself; partly because you will feel satisfied with less, and partly because you will not have the time. You will absorb more Ki and nutrients from well-chewed food.

Living things have more Ki than dead things. Freshness is a good indication of a food's Ki level, assuming it has not been tampered with to give a false impression of freshness. To avoid that pitfall, eat 'organic' as far as possible. Then you know that what you see is what you get. Even when organically grown, if the food looks old and deficient in Ki, then it IS deficient in Ki, meaning less Ki is there for you to extract from it.

Burning food destroys it, leaving proven carcinogenic residues. So avoid burnt or smoked food. If you really want to be healthy, avoid that part of food that has been even lightly browned during cooking. A good motto is: *If it's brown(ed), put it down.*

Water, when heated, exhibits strong Ki, so boiling or steaming your food is good. Steam or boil it just enough to make it easier to eat. Very tough things should be cooked for longer (for example: grains, beans and tough vegetables). More delicate things can be cooked lightly, or not at all.

Avoid consuming too much extremely sweet food too often (sugar and very sweet fruits), as this will overwork your body's ability to maintain correct blood sugar levels. A wealth of information about the effects of sugar has existed for years, so I will not go on about that.

Oils and fats represent the foods that are subject to the worst adulteration. All the necessary trace elements (the good bits) have been removed from commercial oils, and the balance of essential fatty acids has been altered. These essential fatty acids and trace elements are crucial for health, so a low fat or no fat diet can be very detrimental. Lots of bad bits have been added to make your bottle of oil 'neutral' in taste and to extend its shelf life. Try to get oils labelled *unrefined*, extracted from organically grown seeds. Keep your unrefined oil in a sealed dark bottle or container, in a cool place. Light, oxygen and heat destroy natural oils very quickly. For this reason, it is not good to cook with your oils; especially do not fry with them. If you do cook with oil, cook it within water, to avoid raising the oil temperature above boiling point. A temperature more than 15°C above boiling point will tend to destroy most oils. Butter and especially ghee from butter can be cooked at a slightly higher temperature, but even that should be occasional rather than regular.

The closer a food is to its natural state, the better. Eat clear and wholesome food on a day-to-day basis and your Ki will be clear and wholesome. If you eat a cocktail of irradiated chemicals, burnt in your oven, at every mealtime, you will sooner or later feel less than healthy. Some people it is true, get ill even when they consistently eat healthy stuff. But there are countless negative influences bearing down upon us, both from within our psyche and from the environment. It is your constitutional strength which determines your tolerance level for ingesting toxic substances or your ability to survive self-abuse.

In short, eat Ki. Green leafy plants seem to have the most Ki, so eat them in abundance; all the edible parts. Say goodbye to burnt, overcooked, over processed and stale food. Very occasionally enjoy even those things, if it is a choice between isolating your social life, or not.

# Preparing Your Mind

When you put your hands upon someone else's body, the actual mechanics of contact, such as the level of pressure and rhythm of movement, are essential ingredients for good shiatsu. However, this is not the only factor that will have a bearing on how your touch is received. Your state of mind is also very important.

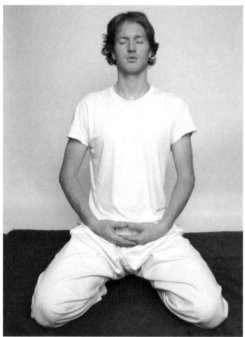

Your attitude to the receiver, your reason for doing shiatsu, your emotional disposition and your ability to remain focused are all critical elements.

## Mental Focus

When applying shiatsu technique, be it a stretch or the application of pressure, you must be aware not to hurt the receiver. Conversely, you should not be so timid with your approach as to lack effectiveness. Often there is a fine line between what is too far a stretch or too much pressure, and what is an insufficient stretch or insufficient pressure. The recognition of this 'line' requires sensitivity; and sensitivity demands a focused mind.

*The photographs show examples of correct postures for seated meditation. All require your back to be fully upright but relaxed.*

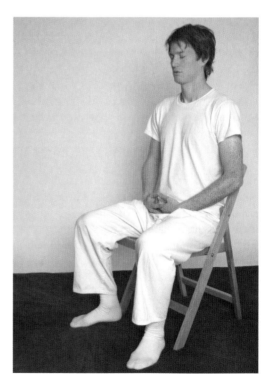

If your mind wanders off whilst giving shiatsu, you will miss the signals that indicate whether or not you should continue to increase or decrease the pressure or stretch. One way of keeping your mind focused is to go slowly and ask the receiver to tell you when you are entering their discomfort zone. However, due to the often extremely relaxing nature of shiatsu, the receiver may put up with moderate pain, and not bother to say anything until their pain is too much to bear. Shiatsu does not need to be painful. If you are alert to the reactions of your touch, you eventually learn to recognize the line between effectiveness and discomfort.

So how can you stay focused? First, you must work on your own body as already described, to ensure you can remain comfortable throughout the shiatsu session. If you are experiencing discomfort, you will be focusing on your own pains rather than the receiver's reactions to your touch. Secondly, you would do well to adopt a method which 'trains' your mind to remain more 'one pointed' and less prone to wandering. There are many meditation, yoga, qigong and 'mindfulness' practices that you could adopt. It is outside the scope of this book to cover these subjects in great depth. However, I will touch upon some basic principles of 'mindfulness' and meditation in this chapter.

**Empathy and Compassion**

In addition to sharpening your mental focus, it is also important to become less self-centred and more caring towards others. If your motivation for giving shiatsu is to genuinely help others, then of course, you will have this quality already. Making a habit of reflecting deeply about the needs and suffering of others will enhance your caring attitude. Please remember that a focused mind does not necessarily mean a compassionate mind. One can focus ones selfishness and hate as easily (if not more easily!) than one can focus compassion. You need compassion to develop empathy; and you need empathy to enhance compassion.

**Mindfulness**

To practice 'mindfulness' means to be constantly aware or 'conscious' of everything we do. It requires us to keep our minds absorbed in the present moment, noticing the detail and nuances of our actions. For example, if we wash a cup with mindfulness, we notice the texture and temperature of the cup. We are aware of how much pressure we are applying to the cup with the cloth or brush. We take note of the speed with which we are conducting the activity, and we become aware of our own physical sensations and thought processes.

The more repetitive or routine the activity, the more likely it is that we will switch to autopilot and allow our minds to dwell elsewhere. This is necessary, to enable us time to make plans or to reminisce. But in our busy, complicated lives we perhaps spend too much time pondering the trivial, dwelling on the past or anticipating future possibilities. We tend to miss a full appreciation of the present, because our minds are perpetually oscillating backwards and forwards through time and space. The past is history and the future is only a possibility. The only 'reality' for us is what our consciousness perceives 'right now'. So, if you wash that cup with your full attention, you will learn a great deal about that cup. Similarly, if you apply your shiatsu touch with your full attention, you will learn a lot about your touch and about how your touch is received. If you make 'mindfulness' a priority and a discipline, you will spend much more time in the 'here and now'. Consequently, you will learn a lot about yourself and about how you interact with others. Your shiatsu will naturally become more sensitive, more empathic and thus, more effective.

Mindfulness develops sensitivity to what is going on within both you and the person or object of your attention. As a result it develops equanimity, because equanimity is the opposite of succumbing to distractions. To illustrate the relevance of this, consider that as a receiver of shiatsu or any other form of bodywork, you will definitely feel more at ease when worked on by a serene and centred person, compared to being treated by someone who is 'spaced out' or clearly preoccupied with some other issue: The former feels great and the latter hurts or irritates you.

One of the easiest ways to practice mindfulness is to observe your own breathing. As long as you are alive you will be breathing, so if breath is the object of your attention, you know you cannot forget to bring it with you. A good technique is to observe the breath as it enters and leaves your nostrils, trying to notice any sensations felt at the point of entry and exit. You may feel this close to the tip of your nose, just inside the nostrils or between your nose and your top lip. Experiment to see which applies to you. Try to register only those sensations felt at this point; in other words, don't follow the breath deeper into the body on the inhalation, or beyond the nose on the exhalation.

Alternatively, be aware of your belly moving slightly in and out as you breathe, relating only to the sensation of your lower belly 'opening' a little as you inhale and 'closing' a little as you exhale. Again, avoid following the breath to see where it goes (although you could do that once or twice as a separate meditation, just to find out!). These techniques are examples of a 'mindfulness of breath' method known as *anapana*.

If you practise breathing with awareness, you will remember to do other things, including shiatsu, with more awareness. Try not to get obsessive about it though, or broadcast the fact that you are doing it. Just quietly continue until it becomes a natural and unobtrusive part of your way of being. You will be pleasantly surprised at the fringe benefits, particularly the way you are able to cope with stress more positively.

**Meditation**

Both mindfulness and anapana are examples of meditation. However, meditation encompasses any method that helps counteract the wandering tendency of our mind so that we can experience things as they really are. It is the term given to those practices that encourage a genuinely objective view of things. Our mistaken view of reality is that we relate to things as if they have some permanent existence, inherently independent of other things. We think of a 10,000 year old stone statue as a stone statue, forgetting that it is only a rock hewn from another rock, and will eventually be eroded into dust. We know this if we are drawn to think about it, but most of the time we do not think this way. We slip into our habit of perceiving such things as absolute unchanging objects. Likewise, we see this person as attractive, or we experience ice cream as delicious. But surely if these qualities were inherent within those things, everyone would experience them in the same way, which of course they do not. The well-known saying: *beauty is in the eyes of the beholder*, illustrates this concept well.

The on-going awareness that things are both forever changing and ultimately interlinked with all other things is the 'reality' that eludes us. We get fleeting moments of 'awakening', but when it really matters, we fall back into our habitually limited way of perceiving things. Take your own experiences as examples: when someone annoys you, you react angrily because they are annoying YOU. Later, you might again remember that the problem was an emotional over-reaction to your own point of view.

Such enslavement to your emotions will affect your shiatsu session. For one thing, it will be difficult to fully concentrate on your receiver if you are still smouldering with anger over some recent incident. Consequently, you might apply a less sensitive touch, thus causing your receiver to suffer unnecessary pain.

The ultimate goal of the full-time meditator is to remain in a state of 'reality awareness' long enough to perceive what life and the universe is all about. However, for full-time and part-time meditators, the short-term benefits consist of:

1. Greater equilibrium and clarity of mind, naturally leading to greater patience and tolerance of others.

2. Less stress, as seemingly stressful things are seen in perspective and therefore reacted to more positively.

3. Better health, because positive mental attitudes can heal physical and emotional problems.

4. Fewer unrealistic expectations of people or things, therefore less disappointments and better relationships.

5. More realistic and positive self-image as our perception of reality broadens and deepens.

*Types of meditation*

There are two broad categories of meditation: *stabilizing* meditation and *analytical* meditation, each of which consists of many methods.

Stabilizing meditations are basically concentration exercises designed to settle the mind into a period of uninterrupted focus on a single point, which is the exact opposite of our usual state of mind, which is forever distracted. Mindfulness practices and concentrating on the breath, both described earlier, are examples of this. Concentrating on a visualized image, a concept, or a mantra are other examples.

Analytical meditations are periods when you draw your mind to consciously reflect upon and analyze a particular concept such as 'emptiness', 'attachment', or the nature of mind itself. The purpose of this method is to gain a conceptual understanding of how things are, to a level that gives you enough clarity to convince you of the true nature of that concept. The process initially involves identifying our wrong conceptions. For example, if we are exploring compassion, we would aim to arrive at some insight about compassion by first eliminating our misconceptions about compassion. Analytical meditation is therefore an intensive inward period of study.

Stabilizing and analytical meditations are usually combined within a single meditation session. For example, as you prepare to meditate on your breathing rhythm, as in 'anapana' (a stabilizing meditation), it is helpful to spend a few minutes clarifying your state of mind and motivation for engaging in that session, which involves analytical thought. During both analytical and stabilizing meditations, your mind will frequently wander, causing you to constantly bring your attention back to your breath, as an anchor for your mind. At times it may be difficult to do this, at which time a return to a period of analyzing your state of mind will help.

During a session of analytical meditation, when you reach the point of intellectual understanding, it is then appropriate to let go of the thought process and focus your attention single pointedly on associated feelings that arise. You will then arrive at a combined intellectual and experiential insight, causing your mind to become 'one' with the object of your meditation. This is unlikely to happen the first time you try it; but with repetition, sooner or later it will.

Your level of success will depend upon your depth of concentration, which comes about through regular practice. Regularity is actually more important than quantity, because your mind is strongly influenced by habitual patterns. If you do it regularly, your mind will come to expect it. This is how both good and bad habits are formed. So how long should the meditation session last? Start with five or ten minutes and build up to thirty minutes; ending your session before fatigue, aching knees and bottoms, and boredom set in. Don't push yourself too hard because as soon as it becomes a burden you won't do it. On some days you will experience more distractions and discomforts while other days you will be serene and focused. This is normal. View the troublesome sessions as opportunities to explore and grow.

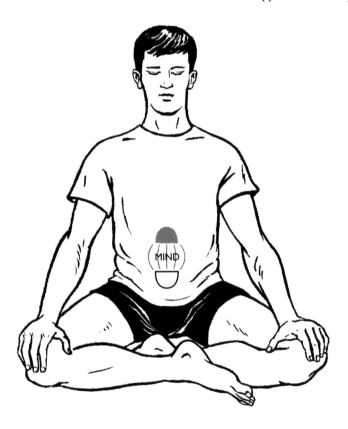

*Active visualizations can help to focus the mind and to prevent sleepiness, restlessness, excitement and other distractions during a shiatsu session.*

Meditation is not essential in order to practise shiatsu on your family and friends, but the more you do, the more it helps. At least employ mindfulness during a shiatsu session. That, I would argue, is essential. Everything else is a (great) bonus.

*Tips for successful meditation*

The biggest obstacles to your meditation practice will be lack of motivation, boredom, sleepiness, restlessness or excitement, discomfort and pain, allowing negative thoughts to proliferate, and lack of input from someone more experienced than yourself. As such, it is recommended that you seek out a good meditation teacher if and when the time comes for you to progress your meditation practice. The qualities you should look for in a teacher include: compassion, knowledge, humility, sincerity, insight, morality and the ability to explain clearly. Your meditation teacher should be someone who thoroughly understands how the mind works; based on his or her own practice. Don't be in any hurry to find that teacher. They will show up when the time is right. Meanwhile, practise what I have suggested in this chapter, and allow your intuition to guide you a little.

*Sleepiness*

- Hold your spine straight, but not tense.
- If your eyes are closed, open them halfway and meditate with your eyes fixed on the floor some way in front of you.
- If you have an unexpected feeling of depression, remember that thoughts and feelings come in waves, so wait for them to pass rather than cling to them.
- If the room is too dark, increase the light slightly.

*Sleepiness antidote visualization*

If the above adjustments fail to stop you wanting to doze off, and you have a visual imagination, try this simple exercise before continuing with your session: Imagine the bottom half of a large hollow white seed about the size of half a tennis ball in your lower belly a couple of inches below your navel. Then picture the top half of a hollow red seed of similar size deep in your solar plexus. Imagine that your mind fills the space between the two seed halves. Now visualize the two seed halves shrinking as they converge just in front of your spine at the level of your umbilicus. As they do so, your mind becomes fully encapsulated within this tiny red and white seed. Now visualize a tube about one fingers width in diameter situated just in front of your spinal column, running from the base of your spine to the top of your head.

Now imagine the seed shoots up through that tube to emerge above the crown of your head. The seed evaporates allowing your mind to expand into, and merge with, a vast empty void. Dwell upon this experience for a few moments before returning to your original meditation.

*Restlessness or excitement*

- Hold your spine straight, but not tense.
- If there is something particularly exciting in your life, reflect upon the fact that excitement is always short term. Feelings such as excitement come in waves so wait for them to pass.
- If your breathing is too quick and too shallow, focus on your lower belly and observe your breathing as if it doesn't belong to you, and notice how it just happens without you having to exert any control over it.
- If the room is too light, decrease the light slightly.

### Excitement antidote visualization

Do the first part of the visualization for sleepiness up to the point where the seed halves shrink and converge with your mind inside it. Dwell for a few moments on the feeling of centredness and groundedness created by the fact that your mind is now snuggled up inside a seed, which is anchored deep in your belly. Then return to your original meditation.

### Discomfort and pain

- Experiment with your position. If you are experiencing lower back pain, sit on a higher and/or firmer cushion. Lean up against something if necessary.

- If there is stress on knee or ankle through as a result of sitting in a cross-legged posture, put cushions under your knees, kneel in seiza (see page 47), or sit on a chair.

- If you are suffering from tension as a result of unresolved worries or anger, use the problem as the focus for your meditation. Also, imagine the pain evaporating from your body with each exhalation.

### Pain antidote visualization

Try the 'body sweep' method: Imagine your consciousness as a gentle shower of cool water washing you down from head to feet, being fully aware of every part of your body as the 'shower' washes over it. Whenever your mind 'washes' into a painful area, imagine the pain is swept away. The hotter your pain, the cooler you should make your 'shower'.

If the pain does not go away, or become acceptable, just observe the pain and try to see it as just another sensation. Alternatively, mentally increase the pain as much as possible before returning to the original pain, which should then seem less intense.

Obviously, if you can neither dispel nor accept the pain, stop the meditation and try again another time.

### Negativity

Negative thoughts that occur as you meditate are not necessarily a problem. It means that your mind is digging up thoughts, feelings and attitudes that are already present. Simply bring your attention back to the breath, then use the negative thought as the object of your meditation.

*Negativity antidote visualization*

Imagine you are sitting neck deep in a tub of warm water. As a negative thought arises, feel it soak out of your body (or out of the red and white seed behind your navel) into the surrounding water. When the water becomes discoloured by your negative thoughts, imagine the water emptying away, so that all those bad thoughts disappear down the drain. The dirtier the water, the better; because it means you are dredging out and expelling more and more negative thoughts. Fill up the tub again, via an imaginary shower pouring onto your head. Repeat until no more negative thoughts arise and the water in the tub remains clean.

When negative thoughts arise during subsequent meditations, do the same visualization and feel you are washing out deeper and subtler layers of mental debris. Avoid trying to repress feelings of negativity, as they will only emerge again later, in an exaggerated form.

What about weird sensations such as your body shrinking or expanding; or your mind leaving your body behind? This is a normal reaction of the mind to meditation, especially in the beginning stages. Therefore, experience them, and then ignore them. They will fade away in due course. These sensations can be quite a 'buzz', but don't get attached to them or wish for them, otherwise they may become major distractions to your focus.

**A meditation checklist**

Make yourself comfortable in your chosen posture.

Check and acknowledge your motivation and goal; it might be simply to calm down, perhaps so you can develop greater 'clarity' when you give shiatsu.

Before you leave your meditation, recall your goal to see whether or not you fulfilled it. For example, have you calmed down (or reached enlightenment)?

Allow much of what you have gained to spill over into your daily life.

Dedicate your efforts and offer your gains to the welfare of others. This really helps link your motivation for meditating with your real reason for doing shiatsu; namely, to help alleviate suffering.

*Should I meditate while giving shiatsu?*

Generally, the best way to apply your mind while giving shiatsu is to be as mindful as possible of everything you do and experience throughout the session; remembering to bring your attention back to the breath when your mind wanders, feeling the slight movement of your lower belly as you breathe.

## Preparing Your Working Environment

This section describes how to ensure optimum conditions for practising shiatsu. Most of what is described here applies equally to activities complementary to shiatsu such as meditation, qigong or yoga.

One of the advantages of shiatsu is that it requires no specialized equipment, other than a mat and a couple of cushions. As such, it is a very portable form of bodywork. However, most professional shiatsu practitioners will rent a room in their local complementary medicine clinic. Some will also work in specialized hospital clinics, alongside Western medical staff. Some will also go to the receiver's place of work or residence. Many practitioners also convert a room in their own residence specifically for giving shiatsu. Those who only practice basic shiatsu techniques on friends and family, will normally visit friends and give shiatsu there, or use a room in their home.

As stated within the section Preparing your Mind (see page 30), it is extremely important to do everything you can to encourage within yourself, a greater equanimity of mind and one pointed mental focus. It makes sense, therefore, to minimize potential stress-inducing situations, especially immediately prior to giving shiatsu. So if you can choose between travelling to someone in the rush hour, or seeing him or her close by, choose the latter. If you have to travel, leave plenty of time and remember to practice 'mindfulness of breath' on the way.

You cannot always choose where to give shiatsu, but if you are in a position to select the optimum location and can influence the ambience of the room, then I offer you a few suggestions.

### The Ambience of Your Shiatsu Room

A separate room used solely for shiatsu is the ideal. This is because the feeling within a defined space, especially an enclosed space, will gradually become influenced by the activities that take place there. If a room is used predominantly for bitter arguments, then a 'bitter argument' atmosphere will permeate the feel of that room. On the other hand, if the room is used solely for shiatsu and activities which prepare you for giving shiatsu (meditation, yoga, qigong and so on), then the room will take on the same peaceful feeling associated with shiatsu.

Creating an ambience of peace and serenity in a room has many clear advantages. Firstly, those who receive shiatsu in that room will react by starting to relax even before you begin working on them. Thus, much of the preparatory work towards reducing their stress will have been fulfilled by the room itself. Secondly, when the positive ambience of the room builds to a sufficient level, the room will become akin to a sanctuary for you. You will find that upon entering the room to give shiatsu, the familiar feeling of serenity associated with that activity in that particular space will over-ride any negative feelings you may have at that time. For example, if you have been working downstairs on a stressful project, or have indulged in some disagreement with your partner, upon entering your 'sanctuary' you will soon feel as if all that is far away. You will in effect, have entered a 'bubble' that seems divorced from the normal stresses of life.

You may have experienced a similar effect when returning to a far away holiday location. Sometimes when you return to somewhere associated with vivid memories, those vivid memories come flooding back, pushing more routine memories and thought processes into the background of your mind. It feels like no significant time has elapsed since you were there before. You seem to have entered a 'bubble' that, in a way, lies outside of time and space.

If you cannot reserve a whole room for shiatsu, try to reserve a space within a quiet room, normally used for something not too frenetic or depressing. A good ambience will still begin to manifest there, but maybe not so quickly or strongly, as the space is not exclusively devoted to shiatsu. If you cannot reserve a corner solely for shiatsu, at least try to give shiatsu in the same place each time. Just going to that familiar location will trigger your mind to switch into shiatsu mode.

**The Contents of Your Shiatsu Room**

Once you have established a location for your shiatsu sessions, what should you put in it? Not much! Material clutter will clutter your mind and that of your recipient. Clutter has its own ambience, and because by definition, there is a lot of it, the ambience tends to be a conflicting mish-mash. All you need is a mat just over 7 feet (2 m) in length and 5 feet (1.5 m) wide, with enough room around it to apply your shiatsu. The shiatsu practitioner will usually use a shiatsu futon that is a mat consisting of two or three layers of compressed cotton or wool, contained within a cotton covering. The futon would thus be about 1–1.5 inches (2.5–4 cm) in depth, compressing down a little with use. For hygiene, place a cotton sheet over the futon and provide a small cloth or some soft paper about the size of a pillowcase to place under their head, particularly for the face down position. Have three or four fairly firm cushions nearby so that you can support the receiver's head and limbs when required.

Lying in a cold room is not much fun for the receiver, so please keep the room warm. In addition, provide a blanket to keep them especially cosy once you have finished. The only other thing you might need is a lightweight cloth about 2.5–3.25 feet (75 cm–1 m) square to place between the receiver's skin and your hands when working on their neck or face, especially if their skin is sweaty or greasy.

Judicious placement of plants will enhance your room. Maybe have a few simple pictures on the wall, but nothing too evocative. You may be tempted to include art and décor that reflects the inner you, but expressing your personality is not the point in this particular room – you have the rest of your house for that. The shiatsu space must be as neutral as possible. Remember, you want to create your 'bubble' to be independent from the rest of your life's ups and downs.

Keep your working space clean, simple and welcoming. Beyond that, you could consider the feng shui (energetic configuration) of the room and either read one of the many books that are available on the subject or contact a feng shui practitioner.

Finally, should you play music while giving shiatsu? Shiatsu does not need the presence of music, so this is very much your choice. However, bear in mind that music can be very evocative. The musical track that may engender serenity in you could remind your recipient of an unhappy or traumatic incident, thus plunging them into depression or grief, so check first that your recipient will find it equally soothing.

**Clothing**

The receiver of shiatsu should remain fully clothed throughout the session. A single layer of cotton or some other natural fibre is best because shiatsu feels better and less obtrusive through a barrier of thin natural fibres. Most synthetic fibres seem to make it more difficult to feel quality of the tsubo. If you apply shiatsu directly to bare skin, it tends to be more superficial in its effect, because the sensation of skin contact distracts the giver from feeling the deeper and subtler presence of Ki. The sensory nerve endings are most prolific on the surface, so a cloth barrier will dampen down the surface tactile sensations and allow the receiver to experience a deeper connection. Although it might seem that a tsubo would be easier to find and feel on bare skin, a little practice through clothing will reveal this to be untrue.

To reduce the likelihood of any sexual connotations arising, it is best to encourage the receiver to wear loose fitting clothing.

For the giver of shiatsu, loose fitting clothing made of a natural fibre is also the preferred option. You need to be able to move around without restriction, and feel well ventilated around your joints. To avoid unnecessary contact between your clothing and the receiver, there should be no dangly bits such as belts, tassels or untucked shirt hems.

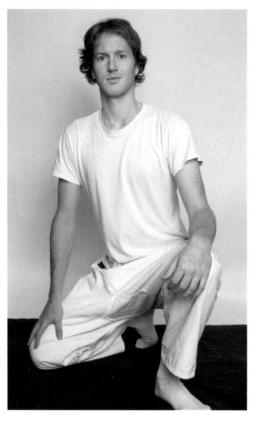

For the same reason that it is not a good idea to make your shiatsu room an extension of your personality, for the shiatsu session, and avoid dressing to make a statement. The more your ego takes a back seat, the easier it is to feel what is happening to the receiver.

*When you are giving shiatsu, wear loose, comfortable clothing made of natural fibres. If the receiver has bare arms or legs, you should wear longer sleeves.*

# CHAPTER 3

# Applying Shiatsu Technique

## The Meaning of Hara

Shiatsu technique should never come from muscular strength, but should utilise gravity wherever possible, which is to say that the giver should lean rather than push or pull. In order to lean correctly, you need to be aware of your centre of gravity, which is located in your belly, or *hara*, as it is called in Japanese (and therefore in shiatsu). If you ensure your movements originate from your hara, then your movements will involve your whole body, thereby utilising the sum total of your body's power. For example, it is well understood in the martial arts that if, when throwing a punch, you focus your mind and breath in the hara and pivot from the lower belly, you will have your whole body weight and power behind that punch. If the punch originates from the shoulder it uses the power of the shoulder only, which has only a fraction of the power that originates from the hara.

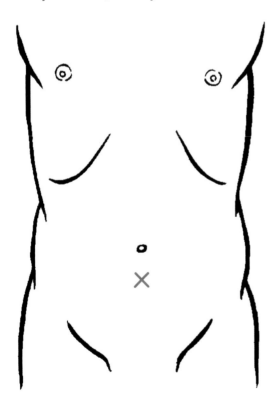

*The location of the tanden.*

Using your hara therefore means that you originate all your movements from your belly, or, to be more specific, from a point just below the navel, which is the body's central pivotal point. This point is known as the *tanden* (or *dantian* in Chinese).

So, whenever you perform a shiatsu technique, you must ask yourself, "from where in my body does the movement originate?"; "where is the root of the technique?". By working backwards from the point of contact you can use 'mindfulness' to detect the source of your pressure or connection. If done correctly, the source will always be found at tanden, in the lower hara. If you want to apply pressure upon the receiver's back with your palm, for example, and you discover that the root of the technique is a push from the shoulders, then you know the technique is not rooted in hara and is therefore ineffective. In fact, it is worse than ineffective, it will create a defensive reaction in the receiver rather than the relaxation response you are trying to achieve.

However, the meaning of hara extends beyond physical movement. It is a term used to illustrate one's ability to achieve. If someone applies himself or herself diligently to fulfil their aim, they are said to have hara. Whether they actually achieve that aim or not is considered a reflection of how strong in hara they are. How one accepts disappointment in not achieving one's aim is also a reflection of hara. That is, the ability to lose with grace, and start all over again with undiminished resolve and effort indicates a good hara.

As such, to have hara means to have the ability to get things done; to not shy away from the difficult and to bounce back after setbacks. So to have a strong hara in shiatsu practice will make your shiatsu more effective on all levels: the techniques will come from a source of relaxed power, and your motivation and ability to keep doing shiatsu will be assured.

Focusing energy in the hara harmonizes the body, mind, emotions and spirit, which enables us to harmonize with our surroundings and react positively to the needs of those receiving shiatsu. When someone is described as 'coming from their hara', the meaning is that they are well grounded, strongly focused and using the maximum potential of their body and mind together.

How do you develop power and focus in your hara? Keep active, stay humble, do lots and lots of shiatsu from your hara and focus your mind frequently upon your hara. You could also practice anapana hara focus (see page 32).

**Why babies give good shiatsu**

If you observe babies as they move, you will see that their movements originate from their centre, their belly. You will never see young babies tensing in the shoulder to push a toy, for example. If you can persuade a baby to crawl about on your back, you will experience the key qualities of shiatsu contact: complete surrender of weight to gravity, giving the quality of 'weight underside'; movements and balance centred and emanating from their belly; an innocent non-analytical acceptance of themselves being there, not invading your space.

A baby's mind, when drawn to an object, will for a while become completely absorbed and preoccupied by that object. During that preoccupied period, their mind is completed 'one-pointed', totally focused. Their consciousness is not yet cluttered and their sense of self is not so separated from their environment. They are thus able to be completely in the present and to relate to the object of their attention as if it is part of themselves.

The shiatsu practitioner tries to recreate those qualities when doing shiatsu. We need to be a little bit 'innocent' to be aware of the receiver's needs; to lose our sense of self in order to really empathize with the other person. Babies empathize perfectly; they are just limited in their variety of means to express that empathy. Adults empathise less perfectly, but have great powers of language to hide their lack of communication abilities.

When we occasionally get a glimpse of what is was like when we were more innocent, we realise just how colourful and rich things really are. To touch another's body with innocence and clarity means we will realise how much more is going on within that person. This is so simple, yet so difficult. It may be a lost art for us adults, but it can be partially regained by observing and contemplating life and by giving attention to how to prepare your body, your mind and your working environment (see Chapter 2).

# Cross Patterning

When we crawl we put one hand forward as we place the opposite knee forward. This leads to a well-balanced and co-ordinated means of getting around. Try crawling by putting the left hand and knee forwards at the same time and see what happens! When you have an opportunity to watch a baby stretch a hand out, notice that their opposite leg moves also. Notice how both the arm and leg movement connects at their hara.

Research has suggested that inhibition of this diagonal limb movement, which is called *cross patterning* or *cross crawling*, inhibits the correct integration of our analytical thought patterns with our more intuitive or experiential thought processes. This implies that it is better for both our physical and mental balance to ensure that when we apply pressure through one hand or forearm during a shiatsu session, we also involve some participation with the opposite leg.

Whether you have your hands on the floor or on a person makes no difference to this principle. Therefore, if you practice this exercise as you apply those shiatsu techniques requiring downward pressure through your hands (see Chapter 4), you will soon get to grips with how to involve and develop your hara as you practise on your friends.

*Try this exercise:*

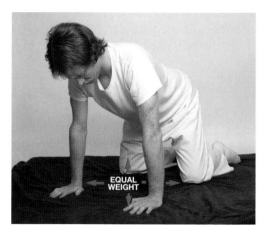

1. Kneel on all fours as if you were about to crawl but with your hands and knees spread a little wider apart and further from your torso, with your weight balanced evenly between your hands and knees.

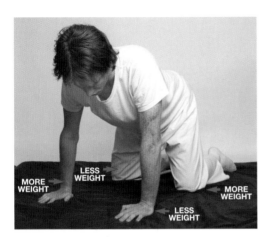

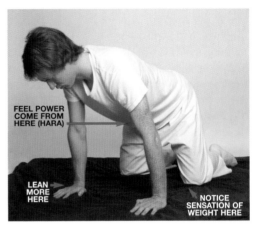

2.  Lean more weight through your right hand by
    shifting your hara slightly towards your right
    hand. Notice that you feel a slight increase in
    weight through your left knee. (If you did not
    clearly feel that diagonal weight distribution
    between hand and opposite knee, lean well
    forwards onto both hands and try lifting your
    left hand off the ground so that the right hand is
    supporting most of your weight. You will notice
    that it is much easier if you also lift your right
    knee off the ground so that it is your right hand
    and left knee supporting your weight).

3.  With your belly completely relaxed and 'open',
    lean more weight through your right hand as you
    take the weight off your left hand, without
    actually lifting your left hand off the ground. Then
    consciously allow your left leg to feel as heavy as
    possible so that your left knee feels more heavily
    pressed into the ground, simultaneously taking
    the weight off your right knee. If you focus your
    attention on your hara as you do this, you will
    feel a sensation of gathering power within your
    hara. Even out the weight distribution between
    all four limbs and repeat this exercise several
    times to appreciate the difference it makes.

What if you lean forwards and apply equal weight through both hands? If you forget about
your legs and concentrate only upon your hands, you will feel the root of the technique
coming more from your shoulders. If you do the same technique but concentrate on the
sensation of connecting to the ground with your knees, you will feel the root of the
technique in your hara.

## Basic Shiatsu Stances

There are several basic positions or stances from which to apply shiatsu technique. Stances fall into three broad categories: Kneeling and Squatting; Sitting; and Standing. Most stances used in technique forms for beginners are drawn from the kneeling and squatting section. More advanced shiatsu techniques sometimes require different stances, but they fall outside the scope of this book.

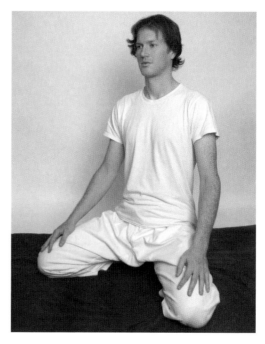

*Wide kneeling.*

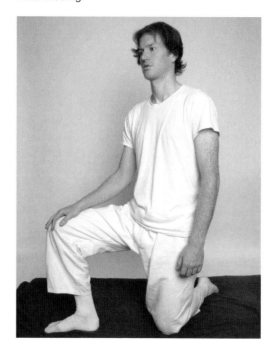

*Half kneeling.*

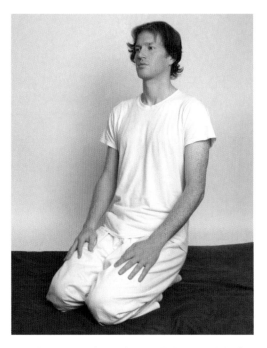

*Kneeling or seiza (sometimes called 'kneel sitting').*

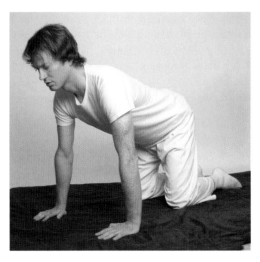

*Prone kneeling.*

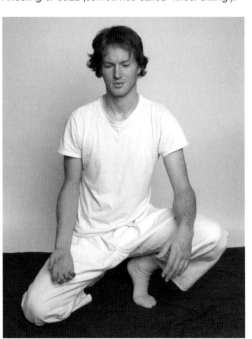

*Squat kneeling.*

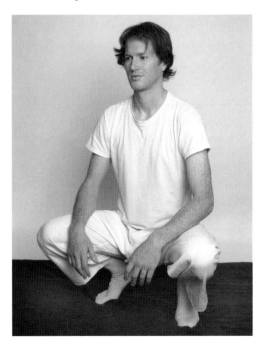

*Squatting.*

## The Correct Posture for Giving Shiatsu

It is important to hold your posture correctly whilst giving shiatsu, as it will make it easier for you to support the receiver's body without fatigue. In addition, it will help you to move around their body more efficiently and generally help your Ki to flow smoothly.

### The basic rules of good shiatsu posture

- Adopt a wide base with your legs, to ensure a low centre of gravity (any of the shiatsu stances described on pages 46–47 will do).

- Keep your hara relaxed and open.

- Look ahead, not down at the receiver (apart from an occasional glance to check that the receiver is comfortable).

- Keep your shoulders relaxed, feeling that the shoulder blades are moving down your back, away from your ears.

- Keep your chest open, without forcing it.

- Feel the back of your neck is open, lengthening and relaxed.

- Imagine that the spaces within the joints of your spine, shoulder, elbows, wrist and fingers are constantly opening as they relax more.

When using your hands to apply shiatsu technique, it is important to ensure that your knee or knees are not positioned between your hands. You need a clear 'view' from your hara to the area you are working on otherwise it is more difficult to apply your weight and to project your Ki or 'intention' from your hara.

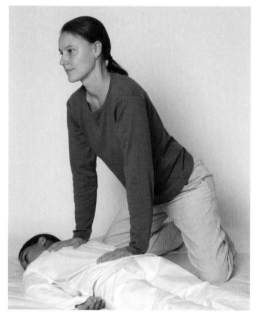

*Correct posture: the head is straight and the eyes are looking straight ahead; the back of the neck is open and lengthening; the shoulders are relaxed, with the shoulder blades descending; the chest is open and the hara is open and relaxed; the base is wide.*

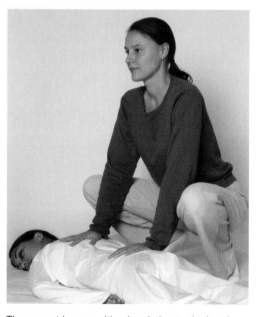

*The correct knee position in relation to the hands while squatting, showing the knees spread to keep the hara open.*

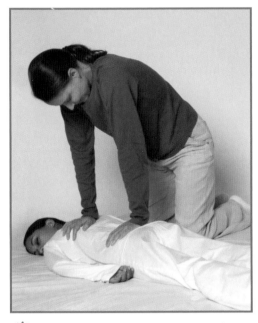

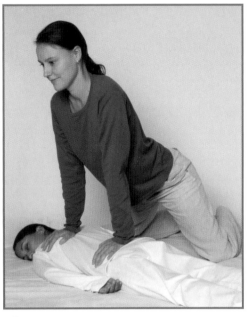

 *Incorrect posture: the giver is looking down, the shoulders are tight, the chest and hara are closed and the base is narrow.*

*Incorrect posture: the lumbar curve is exaggerated, producing potential for weakening the lower back.*

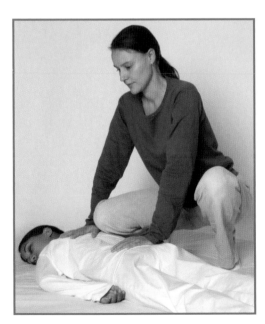

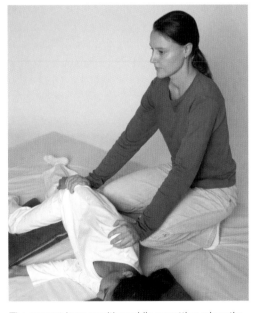

 *Incorrect knee position: the knee between the hands, blocking the hara.*

*The correct knee position while squatting when the knees are used to apply shiatsu technique. The knees are between the hands and the hands are spread wider to ensure balance and control of pressure from body weight.*

## Positioning Your Body in Relation to the Receiver

When giving shiatsu, it is important to make sure that your hara is aligned with the area upon which you are working, or to get as close to that ideal as is practical without sacrificing your comfort. In other words, the more you relax your body when applying pressure, the more your body weight will naturally manifest onto the area you are working and the more your Ki will connect with the receiver.

Connecting your Ki simply means aligning your intention with your action, which is to say taking the most direct route to accomplish your goal. For example, when you are really hungry, you turn to face the food cabinet and walk directly towards it. You would not walk sideways or backwards in a roundabout way to reach the food. Your hara points the way because your hara contains the source of power to reach your goal. In this example, the urge to eat represents your intention. Your mind initially mapped out the route to the refrigerator, and your hara followed that route so that you ended up at the refrigerator door. That one-pointed thought leading to direct action can be considered an example of Ki projection, which is an aspect of what is called *connection*: First you had the idea; the mind then led your Ki towards its goal; your Ki then enabled you to fulfil your goal.

Where it is practical you should align your hara to get the best 'view' down the neck of the tsubo. One way of ensuring your optimum position is to imagine there is a rail running through your hara from the tip of your sternum (breastbone) to your lower belly; then imagine that you have an eye which can move up and down along this rail, but which can only look straight ahead. If you position yourself so that the eye can see down the neck of the tsubo to its base, you will be in a good position to apply technique to that tsubo. More experienced practitioners may not adhere strictly to this rule, but for beginners, it ensures maximum effect whilst keeping the rules simple and minimal.

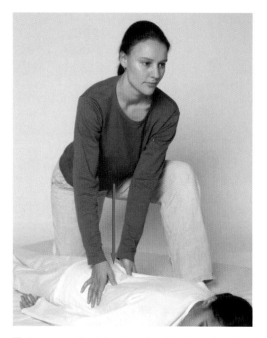

*Tsubo on receiver's body and an imaginary 'eye' positioned on the giver's hara, aligned such that the eye can see directly down the neck of the tsubo.*

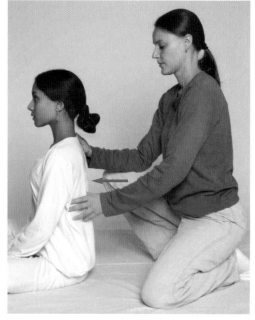

*The hara aligned with the area of the body upon which you are working.*

# Applying the Techniques

No special equipment is required to give shiatsu – different parts of your body are the only tools you need to apply the techniques. The part you use depends upon the type of connection and pressure you wish to give. For beginners, open palms, thumbs, forearms and knees are the predominant 'tools'. Experienced practitioners will sometimes use their hands in different ways to apply specialized techniques.

### Palm Techniques

The palms are the main tool used for shiatsu on family and friends. Although less specific than the use of thumbs or fingertips, the palms have a more soothing quality. If a friend is distressed, we are naturally inclined to place a palm on their shoulder as a gesture of support, rather than lean a thumb into their back! The palms are icons of interpersonal communication, as illustrated by the gesture of shaking the hand of someone you meet.

The Heart Protector channel (sometimes called the Pericardium channel) terminates in the palm (see page 175 for an illustration of the Heart Protector channel, and page 174 for a description of the Heart Protector's function). One of the subtle functions of the Heart Protector, on the psychological level, is that it enables us to share warmth, rapport and close communication with another individual. In a way, it acts as the avenue for spreading our consciousness throughout our body. The fact that the Heart Protector flows into the palm means that when we touch someone, we can give a 'conscious' touch. It enables us to transmit friendliness.

The Ki of the Heart Protector (your warm, supportive, healing quality) exits the body from the centre of the palm, at a point called Heart Protector 8 or 'Laogong', located at the place where the tip of your middle finger lands when you make a fist.

The whole surface of your palm should be kept in full contact with the recipient so that your hand can mould around the contours of their body. The palms will therefore lie more flat on their back, or curl to envelope an arm or an ankle. The palms and fingers must remain relaxed. The arms should remain outstretched, but with the elbows unlocked.

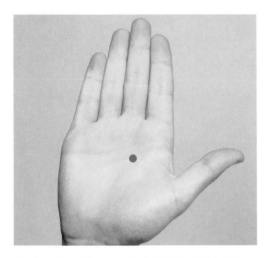

The location of Laogong in the palm of the hand.

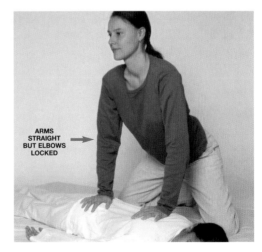

ARMS STRAIGHT BUT ELBOWS LOCKED →

Applying palm pressure the receiver's back with the elbows outstretched but unlocked.

When closer body contact is required, it may be necessary to have the arms angled 90 degrees at the elbow, with the knee or inner thigh supporting your upper arm. However, this will cause a slight reduction in the connection of Ki flow between your hara and your palm (see right).

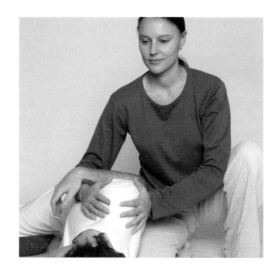

### Support hand technique

Keep both hands separated but in contact with the receiver. This is the most basic, yet most important therapeutic shiatsu technique. It enables the giver to 'listen' with one hand while the other hand is engaged in techniques to tonify, calm or disperse Ki. The listening hand is often called the support hand or the mother hand, while the active hand is sometimes called the working hand or the child hand. When tonifying, the working hand should be applied at right angles to the area of contact. Dispersing techniques are any active techniques such as shaking, rubbing, circling and especially stretching. Calming is an attitude rather than a technique: if you are very calm and composed, that calmness will influence the receiver's Ki at the point of contact.

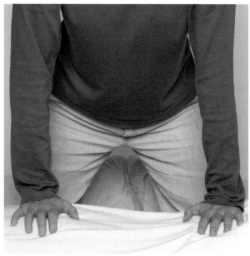

*The support hand is on the receiver's body, and the working hand is applied at right angles to the area of contact.*

### Palm overlap technique

Place one hand on top of the other. This technique can be used when a malleable 'wave like' action is required. It is typically used directly on the receiver's belly for alleviating digestive stagnation.

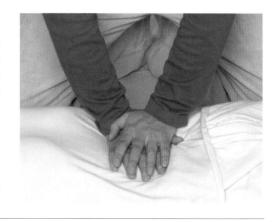

*In palm overlap technique, the hands are placed one on top of the other.*

*Circular rotations*

With one palm moulded into the contours of the shoulder blade, buttocks or sacrum, firmly rotate the connective tissues over the underlying bone rather than merely scrubbing the surface. The other palm can be positioned either nearby on the body, or on top of the other hand. Rotations are especially effective for relieving muscular tensions around the shoulder blades, or for stimulating warmth in the pelvic region when applied to the sacrum.

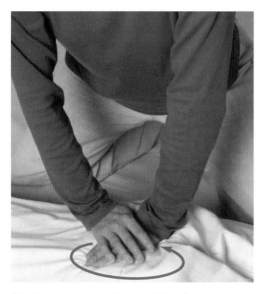

*For circular rotations, the giver's hands can be placed one on top of the other.*

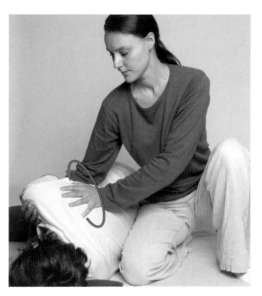

*An alternative method for circular rotations involves the giver placing one hand on the receiver's shoulder and the other on the shoulder blade.*

*Shaking*

Place the palm in the same way as you did for rotations, but shake it instead of rotating it. The effects are similar.

*Grasping*

One hand clasps the limb for support, while the other moves along the limb. Also, both hands can clasp a limb as you stretch that limb away from the space between your hands.

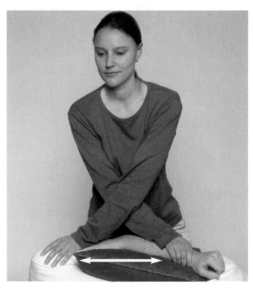

*For grasping, the receiver is in side position. The giver has his arms crossed and both hands clasp the receiver's arm.*

*Double palm squeezing*

Interlock your fingers and apply a squeezing movement simultaneously with the heels of both hands. This method is useful for squeezing the muscles either side of the lumbar spine, from the kidney region down to the pelvis.

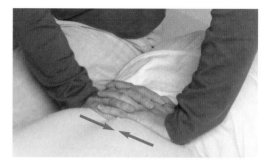

*With the receiver in prone position, the giver is applying double palm squeezing to the lower back with the heels of both hands.*

*Palm off the body method*

Holding the palms a few inches away from the body has a warming effect if the giver is relaxed and centred. This method is especially effective when applied over the face, which can be a pleasant way to conclude a session. When Ki sensitivity is developed, local excess or deficiency of Ki can be clearly assessed using this technique.

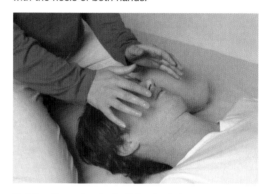

*Holding the palms just off the body has warming effect.*

## Thumb Techniques

The thumb is the classic tool of shiatsu and some styles of shiatsu use the thumb almost exclusively, although this is very limiting; one tool rarely suffices for a range of variable situations.

As the thumb is shorter and thicker than the other fingers, having only one interphalangeal joint instead of two, it is the strongest individual digit. Therefore, strong pressure can be applied and sustained by the thumb if necessary. The ball of the thumb is used for most applications, although the area near the tip can be employed when working with light pressure between small muscle groups such as exist in the neck

Some people have very flexible thumbs that bend backwards when pressure is applied through them. If your thumb is of this type you run the risk of overstraining the interphalangeal joint and should minimize the use of your thumbs and make more use of the palms or fingers.

It may be that you will have difficulty keeping your thumbs straight, allowing them to buckle at the interphalangeal joint. If you apply strong pressure like this over a period of time, you will damage your thumb joints. Even light pressure given with buckled thumbs is discouraged. This is because Ki moves in straight lines or smooth curves; it does not make sharp right-angled turns. Therefore, if your thumbs are buckled, you will feel less and give less through them.

There are two main methods for supporting your thumb pressure; the open hand and the closed hand methods. Two other variations of thumb application, the thumb adjacent technique and the thumb overlap method, enable greater pressure to be applied. However, such heavy pressure is unnecessary if your awareness and Ki is accurately focused on the kyo areas.

*Open hand method*

For maximum stability it is preferable to have your thumb in contact with the receiver's body and your other four fingers spread lightly in contact, as shown right.

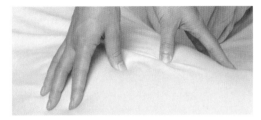

*Open hand method applied to the receiver's back.*

*Closed hand method*

Alternatively, the four fingers can be formed into a fist so that the thumb can be supported against the index finger. This method is a useful alternative for those with hyper-mobile interphalangeal joints, but it does sacrifice stability compared to the open hand method.

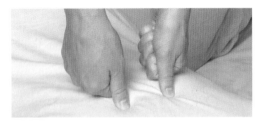

*Closed hand position with fists supporting thumb.*

*Thumb adjacent technique*

Thumbs are placed side by side, either in open hand or closed hand configuration.

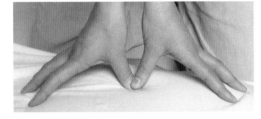

*Thumb adjacent method with open hand support.*

*Thumb overlap method (with open hand support)*

One thumb is placed directly on top of the other. The weight is given more through the top thumb, allowing the lower thumb to be more passive. The open hand method with fingers spread lightly to each side can be used for support.

*Thumb overlap method with open hand support.*

*Thumb overlap method (with closed hand support)*

As described above, one thumb is placed directly on top of the other, but a closed fist resting on the receiver's body achieves support.

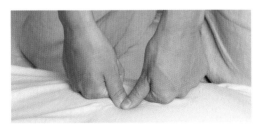

*Thumb overlap position with closed hand support.*

## Finger Techniques

The fingertips are excellent tools for sensing the Ki within the channels and feeling other subtle activity registering near the surface of the receiver's body. This is because the fingers have a rich supply of sensory nerve endings. Please make sure you keep your fingernails and thumbnails short. Fingernails have no sensory nerve endings, so you will feel nothing through them. However, the receiver will certainly feel something if you dig your fingernails into their body!

### Three- or four-finger method

Using the middle three fingers simultaneously is a good method for tracking along a Ki channel to find the kyo and jitsu discrepancies within that channel. Professional shiatsu practitioners also use three fingers of each hand to feel for kyo/jitsu patterns in the hara. It is also an excellent technique for tonifying the spaces between the ribs, close to the breastbone (sternum). Placing all four fingers of one hand on the receiver's mid or upper back and circling or shaking them can be an effective way to disperse tension in the intercostal muscles between the ribs.

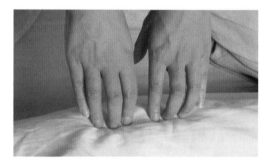

*Three fingers of each hand tracking the Stomach channel in the thigh.*

A two-handed version of the four-finger method can be used to disperse tension in the muscles close to the spine, using a to and fro 'push-pull' movement known as *kenbiki*. Your thumb should be relaxed and your fingers strong (constant practice will quickly strengthen them). Like all shiatsu techniques, the movement must originate from your hara, with a sense of connection to tanden. This will prevent fatigue and tension accumulating in your wrist.

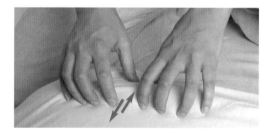

*Four fingers of both hands doing 'kenbiki' technique for dispersing the muscles close to the spine.*

### Index finger method

This technique is a useful alternative to the thumbs for people with hyper-mobile thumb joints. It is particularly useful for applying pressure to the side of the receiver's nose.

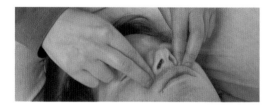

*Index finger method.*

### 'Vee' finger technique

The middle and index fingers are lightly pressed simultaneously either side of the spinal column in small children.

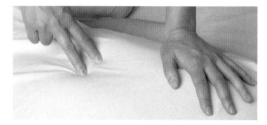

*'Vee' finger technique.*

**Finger/Thumb Combination Techniques**

*Dispersing claw technique*

The thumb and fingers are slightly curled to form a claw. The claw is then pressed into the body and quickly withdrawn, as if pulling strands out of the body. In reality, excess Ki is being pulled out of the area being worked on. This technique is specific for pulling accumulated Ki (jitsu) from the shoulder blades or buttocks. It is never to be used on kyo areas, as this will make the already deficient area much more so.

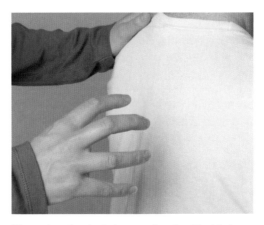

*Dispersing claw technique on the shoulder blade.*

*Tonifying claw technique*

This hand position is similar to the dispersing claw technique, except that the fingers and thumbs are less spread. The thumbs are completely straight and the fingers are only slightly curved. This technique is particularly good for working down both sides of the spine at the same time, either in the sitting or facedown positions. The thumb is positioned to one side of the spinal column and the fingers are positioned on the opposite side

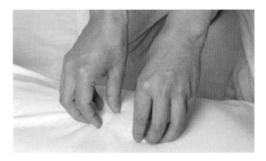

*Tonifying claw technique using both hands down centre of the back with the receiver in facedown position.*

*Dragon's mouth technique*

Spread your thumb and index finger wide. Contact is applied through the 'vee' shape. The 'dragon's mouth' is used primarily to apply pressure to the occiput. Both hands can be used together to apply pressure to the waist in the side position. The Dragon's Mouth can also be applied to the limbs; in which case the fingers are bent rather than straight, to give a stronger contact.

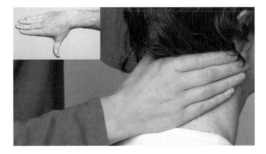

*Dragon's mouth hand configuration.*

*Baby dragon's mouth technique*

Make a fist, but with your thumb and index finger positioned as shown right. Like the tonifying claw technique, this technique is used mainly for working down both sides of the spine at once (see right), in sitting, side and sometimes face down position.

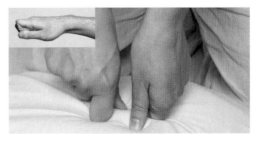

*Baby dragon's mouth hand configuration.*

## Other Hand Techniques

Other hand techniques are occasionally used to disperse jitsu areas, as well as to increase blood and lymph to the skin and superficial muscles. These techniques have a very localised effect and are therefore subsidiary to the mainstream techniques. Used by themselves they are fairly superficial in effect. Even so, beginners should not apply these techniques to chronically ill people, because they will be weakened still further if their Ki is dispersed too much. Therefore, except in specialized circumstances, these techniques are best reserved as useful adjuncts for loosening up robust recipients, especially in the sitting position.

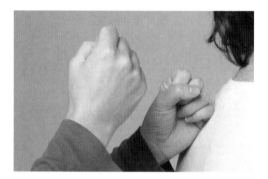

*Pummelling with loose fists.*

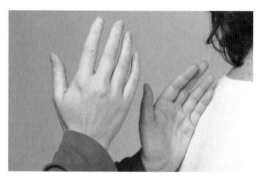

*Loose finger chopping.*

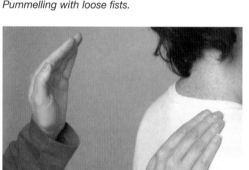

*Palm cupping.*

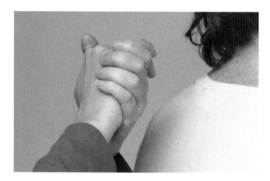

*Double hand cushioning.*

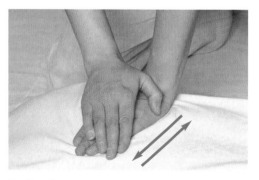

*Rocking (very gentle rocking is suitable for recipients depleted in Ki, but more vigorous rocking should be reserved for those of a more jitsu profile).*

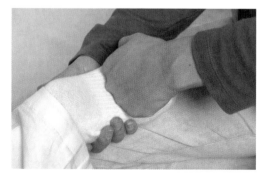

*Knuckle rolling applied to the receiver's feet in prone position.*

## Forearm and Elbow Techniques

The area of your forearm close to your elbow can be used to apply strong pressure to the back, hips and feet. The forearm, or both forearms together, should be applied only after the area to be worked on has been palpated by the hands. This is because they are far less sensitive than the hands. If you attend a beginner's course, the teacher will almost certainly say, "if you haven't got forearms, use two!" This must be the most overused wisecrack in the world of shiatsu!

### *Single forearm technique*

One forearm applied to the sole of the foot gives a great feeling of ironing out tension in the foot. Make sure your wrist is totally relaxed. As usual, all the pressure must come from leaning, never pushing.

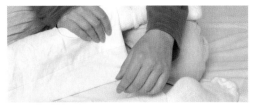

*Single forearm technique applied to the sole of the foot.*

### *Double forearm technique*

Use both forearms together on the back, to stretch the back. Forearms can also be used on the buttocks or thighs.

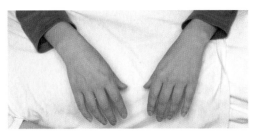

*Double forearm technique applied to the back.*

### *Elbow technique*

The elbows can be used on the same areas of body as the forearms when a stronger and more focused pressure is required. An acutely flexed elbow gives the strongest pressure, which in most cases is too much. A more open elbow joint angle gives a more comfortable pressure. The pressure can therefore be varied according to the angle of the elbow joint. It is essential to keep the wrist relaxed and fist open. You should not use your elbow until you have developed a high level of sensitivity with other 'tools' such as your palms.

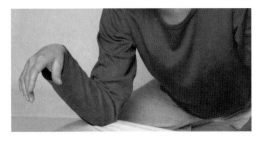

*Elbow technique applied to the back at an acute angle.*

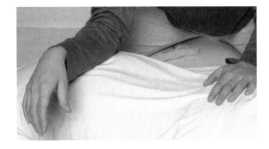

*Elbow technique applied to the back at an open angle.*

## Knee Techniques

Although you can develop great knee sensitivity by constantly practising techniques with them, they will never be as sensitive as your hands. Consequently, use them with discretion only on areas that have been previously checked by your hands. Your knees can be applied individually or together; and you can give very firm pressure with them if necessary.

Keep both hands on the receiver's body so that your body weight is supported through your hands rather than through your knees. In other words, your hands must be positioned so that you can instantly remove them if necessary, to ensure the receiver's comfort and your own stability.

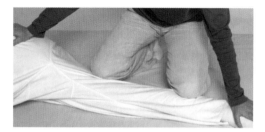

*The knees on the inner thigh in side position.*

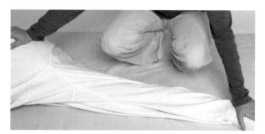

*The weight is taken through the hands as the knees are lifted off the thigh.*

## Feet Techniques

Your feet can be a very useful tool for shiatsu. Although less sensitive than the hands, they can give a very 'earthy' quality to a session. This is because they spend most of their time in contact with the ground. If you intend to use your feet for shiatsu, you should walk around in bare feet as much as possible to give them an even greater earthy quality. Qigong will give your feet a feeling of connection with your tanden (your lower belly), improving your balance. You can further enhance this quality by imagining your feet are being filled from tanden with sand or some other heavy substance.

The feet can be used to stand on the receiver's ankles, which helps tonify the kidneys. However, you must check that the ankles are flexible enough. Test by applying light downward pressure onto their heels with your hand. If the space between their instep and the floor disappears, and there is no pain in their knee, then the technique is considered safe. Do not stand on their heels. Your toes should be on their ankles and your heels should be on their soles. Get feedback from the receiver at every stage.

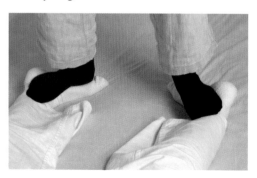

*The feet can be used to stand on the ankles.*

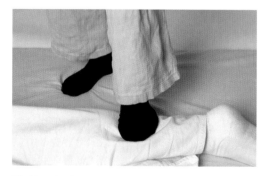

*Shaking the foot on the calf muscles. Avoid the knee joint.*

# Offering Maximum Support and Connection

### The Four Levels of Support

Support has four aspects or meanings within the context of shiatsu, called *levels of support*.

The first level of support is to assist your recipient rather than impose yourself and your shiatsu upon them, so they will feel secure, trusting and be at ease. If you are cold, indifferent or overbearing, they will not drop their barriers and may even feel aggressive towards you. Therefore, the first level of support is one of 'supportive attitude'.

The second level of support is to ensure physical stability for the receiver, so that they remain in position when you are working on them. The most stable position for the recipient is to lie flat on the floor, either face up or face down. In this position no muscular tension is required to offset the effect of gravity, which is forever trying to pull us onto the floor anyway. Ensuring your recipient's physical comfort also falls into this second level of support. In this regard, the judicious use of cushions for comfort and support can make a great deal of difference. For example, when they are in the face down position you might want to place cushions under their feet to support their instep, especially when applying techniques to their lower legs.

Sometimes, lying face down can aggravate a weak or tender lower back, because the lumbar spine feels compressed. Placing one or two cushions under the receiver's belly to 'open' their lower back can sometimes offset this.

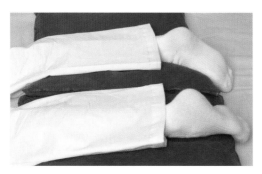

*Cushions placed under the receiver's insteps when face down can make stiff insteps or knees more comfortable.*

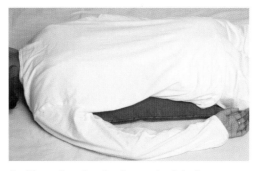

*Cushions placed under the receiver's belly when face down may help relieve those with lower back problems.*

Perhaps the biggest problem with the face down position is that many people cannot get their neck into a comfortable position. Lying with the head turned to one side is the most relaxing position if the neck is flexible enough. Those with stiff necks often try to lie with their nose on the mat, which even if they somehow manage to breathe, will eventually cause fatigue in their upper back and neck. People with slightly stiff necks may still be able to lie with their head turned to one side if they place their arms on the floor beyond their head. However this does make it more difficult for the giver to get into the Bladder channel tsubos around the nape of the neck and upper back. From that point of view, it is better if the receiver has their arms down by their sides, but their comfort is the prime consideration. If it is uncomfortable for them to lie with the neck turned to one side or the other, try placing a cushion underneath the shoulder on the same side that the head is turned, in order to take the strain off their neck. For those who can afford it, there is a system of moulded body support cushions designed to provide maximum comfort for the receiver, particularly when they are lying face down.

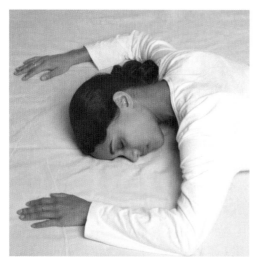

*Some receivers find it more comfortable to position their arms beyond the head when lying face down.*

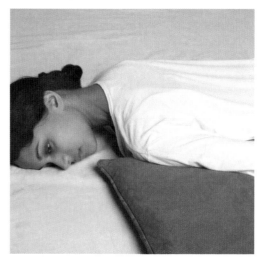

*For a stiff neck when turning to one side in the face down position, place a cushion under the corresponding shoulder.*

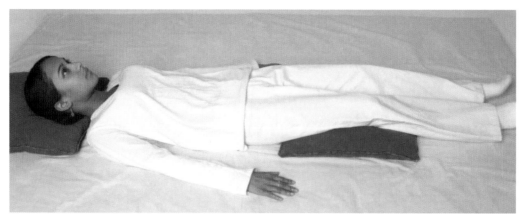

*A cushion placed under the knees can ease knee and lower back problems, while a cushion under the head can help relieve the pain of a stiff neck.*

When lying face up, some receivers, particularly those with certain back problems, will feel more comfortable with cushions placed behind their knees. Those with round shoulders and / or stiff necks may be more comfortable with a cushion or pillow under their head. However, some people actually prefer to lie completely flat on their back, with no supporting cushions.

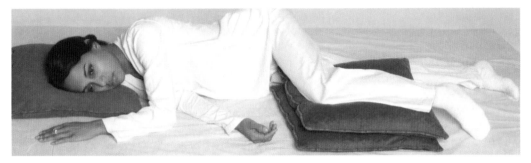

*A cushion placed under the receiver's head and knee when she is in side position can make the hip and head more comfortable and will help prevent over-straining the neck.*

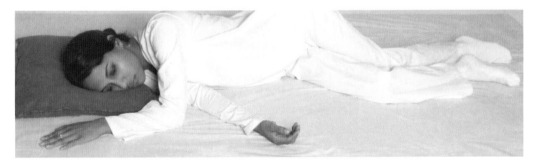

*Alternative leg position, especially good for those who tend to collapse onto their front.*

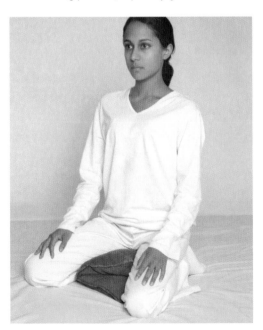

In the side position you should support the receiver's head with a pillow and position their legs in such a way as to prevent the receiver from rolling onto their belly. Sometimes it helps their comfort to have a cushion under their knee.

In the sitting position, some receivers prefer to kneel while others prefer to sit cross-legged. You can make kneeling more comfortable for some people by placing a firm bolster between their legs to take the pressure off their thighs and insteps. However, this could make the comparatively tall receiver too high for you to apply shiatsu from kneeling or squatting and too low to approach them from standing.

*A bolster between the legs makes kneeling more comfortable.*

If the receiver prefers to sit cross-legged, they will naturally be lower to the ground, which is an advantage for the smaller practitioner. Some people cannot sit comfortably cross-legged because their pelvis tilts too far back, causing lower back fatigue, in which case seat them on a thick, firm cushion or a firm foam block of 2.5–6 inches (6–10 cm) deep. This will tilt their pelvis forwards and take the strain off their lower back.

The third level of support is the supportive touch. The receiver may react defensively if you push or press, but by initiating your movement from hara, and leaning rather than pushing, your touch will be welcomed rather than repelled. The recipient will therefore open and relax rather than tighten and close.

Finally, the fourth level of support is to be accessible if the receiver needs to clarify any after effects arising out of their shiatsu session, in which case a supportive dialogue will put their mind at ease. This is more relevant for professional practitioners who are treating people with more serious problems. At this grass-roots level, where you will be giving general shiatsu for stress reduction, it is rare to invoke any uncomfortable after-effects.

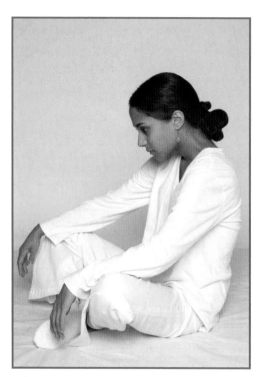

 *Tilting back in the cross-legged position can be uncomfortable.*
**STOP**

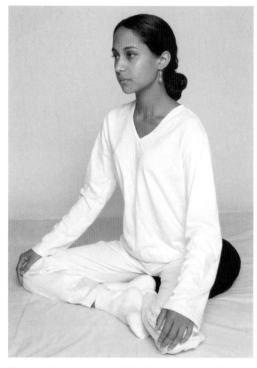

*The receiver more upright in the cross-legged position, with a firm cushion under her buttocks.*

## Two-hand Connection

The techniques that have the most profound effects upon the receiver's Ki are those that involve having both hands in contact with the receiver's body. The hands are your most sensitive Ki imbalance detectors and Ki projectors. Therefore, it stands to reason that two hands should be twice as effective as one hand. Two hands are even more effective if they are separated while in contact, rather than one overlapping the other. If performed correctly, the two hands separated method will result in the receiver experiencing both places of contact as one single unified area. This gives a deep feeling of the whole body being involved in the process. The body and mind will 'open' and relax because the person's parasympathetic nervous system will be activated. Conversely, a single point of contact gives only a localized soothing or dispersing effect, which may be appropriate for more superficial, local relief of pain or stiffness, but does not have the same potential for addressing the Ki at the core level.

To get away from a purely mechanical touch and develop the most conscious touch, you should do the following:

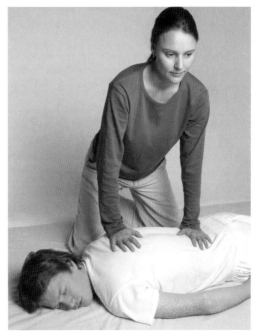

With two hands separated and in contact with the receiver, focus your mind on your hara rather than on your hands.

- With two hands separated and in contact with the receiver, focus your mind on your hara rather than on your hands.

- Sense that your hands begin in your hara. You can do this by focusing on your inhalation and exhalation, as if you are breathing through your lower belly (see page 31).

- Tune into the sensation that your arms and hands are 'breathing' in unison with, and as an extension of, your hara.

- Now feel as if your total body breathing includes the part of the receiver's body that lies between your hands.

Once you have achieved this, you will experience both yourself and your recipient as part of the same circuit. If your focused awareness can be sustained, you may sense the receiver's whole body as one integrated breathing, living unit. You might even feel yourself 'as one' with the recipient. A very sensitive practitioner can sometimes sustain this sensation when one hand is stationary and the other hand is moving, which greatly enhances the quality of continuity.

This level of awareness takes a considerable amount of practice so do not despair if nothing happens when you try this for the first few times. For beginners, the very profound benefits of two-hand connection will still be there whether or not you, the giver, actually experience these Ki sensations.

## Two-hand Connection Along a Ki Channel

When working to balance kyo-jitsu within a Ki channel, two-hand connection is essential. This level of work may begin early on in shiatsu training, but will become more central to your shiatsu practice as your experience progresses.

In the practical application of two-hand connection, one hand will assume a more supportive or yin role and the other a more active or yang role. The support or yin hand is sometimes called the 'mother hand' or 'listening hand', whereas the active or yang hand is often called the 'child hand' or the 'working hand'. In either role, the part of the hand used can be the palms, thumbs or fingertips. However, the support hand mostly makes use of the palm. The basic technique is as follows:

1.  *The support hand remains stationary on one part of the Ki channel, preferably a more jitsu part, while the working hand works down another part of the channel.*

2.  *If the working hand is on a jitsu area, you either move it onto a kyo area or you apply techniques to disperse the blocked Ki from the jitsu area. (A dispersing technique is any active technique such as shaking, circling, stretching or contracting followed by stretching). Meanwhile, the support hand 'listens' for the effects generated by the activity of the working hand.*

3.  *If the working hand is on a kyo area, apply stationary perpendicular pressure (pressure applied at right angles to the area of contact) and wait for a reaction between the two hands. Often you will sense some activity in the kyo area through the working hand, or in the jitsu area through the support hand. The best result is to feel both, which indicates that the two areas are interrelating. A feeling of 'opening', then 'filling up' in the kyo area or tsubo is ideal, especially if accompanied by a feeling of yielding and emptying in the jitsu area.*

4.  *If no response is felt after about 30–60 seconds, you can allow your support hand that is over the jitsu area to become the working hand and apply some dispersing techniques to that jitsu area. Sometimes this will 'shake up and wake up' the blocked Ki, inspiring some of it to move towards the kyo area.*

By working in this way, you are coaxing the Ki to move from where it exists in excess to where it is deficient. If you can move the Ki from a jitsu area into a kyo area, as in step 3 described above, you will have succeeded in dispersing a jitsu area or tsubo as the direct result of tonifying a kyo tsubo. This is the best, deepest, most long lasting and painless method. It is much better than just dispersing the jitsu without addressing the kyo. If you get the desired response during step 3, dispersing techniques such as shaking, circling and stretching are superfluous. However, if you do not get the desired response, you can use the dispersing techniques to coax things along a bit, as in step 4.

So, in effect, two-hand connection is the method to draw Ki along the Ki channels, in so doing, smoothing out the Ki distortions within that channel; the effect of which will spill over into other channels, helping to regulate the body/mind functions in general.

*Moving the Ki from the Hara*

Because your storehouse of Ki is within the hara, the object of shiatsu is to get your receiver's Ki to move from their hara through the limbs and into their hands and feet. For this reason, the support hand should be positioned closer to the centre of their body as the working hand gradually progresses away from the support hand and thus away from the centre of the body. In other words, the hands should start closer together and move apart rather than start apart and move together. Why? Imagine you are trying to keep track of a friend in a railway station bustling with people. It is easier to start off together and maintain visual contact as your friend moves progressively further away, compared to trying to pick her out of a crowd from a distance. Likewise, your hands can maintain Ki connection between themselves more easily if they start off closer together than from far apart.

Consequently, we have some rules regarding two-hand connection:

1. The support hand rather than the working hand should, where possible, be positioned closer to the centre of the receiver's body.

2. The working hand should move away from the support hand, not towards it.

3. No more than one joint should be between the support and working hands. This is because joints interfere with clear communication between your hands. You can feel the Ki with one joint in the way, but it is very difficult with two joints in the way.

4. The support hand and working hand should be applied with equal awareness. This ensures total communication and awareness of Ki flow between your hands. This is sometimes interpreted as equal pressure. For beginners, equal pressure is quite a good rule, although as your sensitivity develops, the actual equanimity and level of pressure becomes less important.

## Maintaining a Fluent Continuity of Technique

Adequate connection and support within good shiatsu technique will enable the recipient to experience a feeling of integration throughout their body and mind as long as the giver of shiatsu can maintain continuity. In order to achieve that:

1. Apply your shiatsu session in a co-ordinated flowing manner rather than as a disjointed amalgam of random techniques. The technique sequences (pages 71–127) exist to give you a framework to work within. If you keep practising these technique sequences, your mind will become free of the burden of deciding what to do next. Later on, when you are fluent in technique, you can be much more spontaneous and innovative in your shiatsu sessions.

2. Each technique should be a logical extension of the previous one, and wherever possible, contact should be maintained as your hands glide from one position to the next. So keep your hands in contact even when moving down their arm, leg or back, or changing technique. Making and breaking contact continuously will inhibit the receiver's ability to deeply relax, because they will be unsure where your hand will land next.

The next four chapters will deal specifically with a detailed description of how to apply fluent technique sequences correctly. Each technique will be described in detail, along with precise instructions on how to move efficiently from one technique to the next.

## Contraindications to Shiatsu

Because this is a book for beginners and meant only as a supplement to personal or class instruction from an experienced shiatsu teacher, you should only practise the techniques described in the following chapters on people who are fit and well. Do not practice on people who have problems such as:

• osteo-arthritis • rheumatoid-arthritis • high or low blood pressure • contagious diseases • fever • cancer • heart disease • life threatening conditions generally.

You should also limit your shiatsu by avoiding parts of the receiver's body affected by:

• varicose veins • burns • open sores • broken bones • bruises.

You should also avoid working directly on painful areas, such as tight or pulled muscles, ligament injuries or joint tenderness. Work around these areas instead.

In addition, do not give shiatsu to women during their first three months of pregnancy. Thereafter, for the remainder of the pregnancy you should avoid giving shiatsu below the knee. This is because there are several tsubos in this area that can initiate a miscarriage.

Your shiatsu mantra is: "*If in doubt, don't do it*". If you attend a proper series of shiatsu classes, you will learn when you can and cannot give shiatsu to people with certain problems. A book can never be a substitute for the one-to-one advice supplied by a personal teacher with whom you can discuss situations that arise.

## The Well-prepared Session

### Dressing for Shiatsu

- Shiatsu not only feels better when received through a single layer of cotton or other natural fibre, but such clothing will also enable the giver to move freely and to feel well-ventilated around the joints.

- Clothing that is free of any tassels, belts, etc., helps avoid any unnecessary contact between giver and receiver.

- Long sleeves are preferred as direct contact with the skin can distract the giver from sensing the presence of Ki.

### Mental Preparation

- The giver has warmed up physically and is now prepared for moving freely around the receiver at floor level.

- The giver's state of mind has an important bearing on the receiver. Qigong exercises have helped ground his body and clear his mind ready for a focussed session of shiatsu.

### Correct Posture for Giving Shiatsu

- The giver is looking ahead rather than down at the receiver.

- His neck, shoulders and chest are open and relaxed.

- His knees are spread to keep the hara relaxed and open.

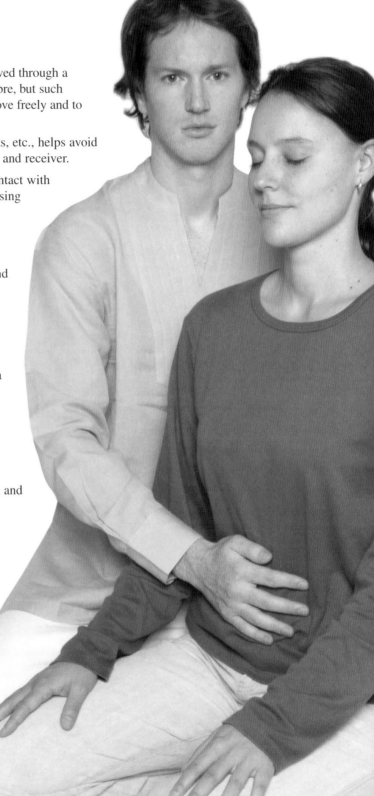

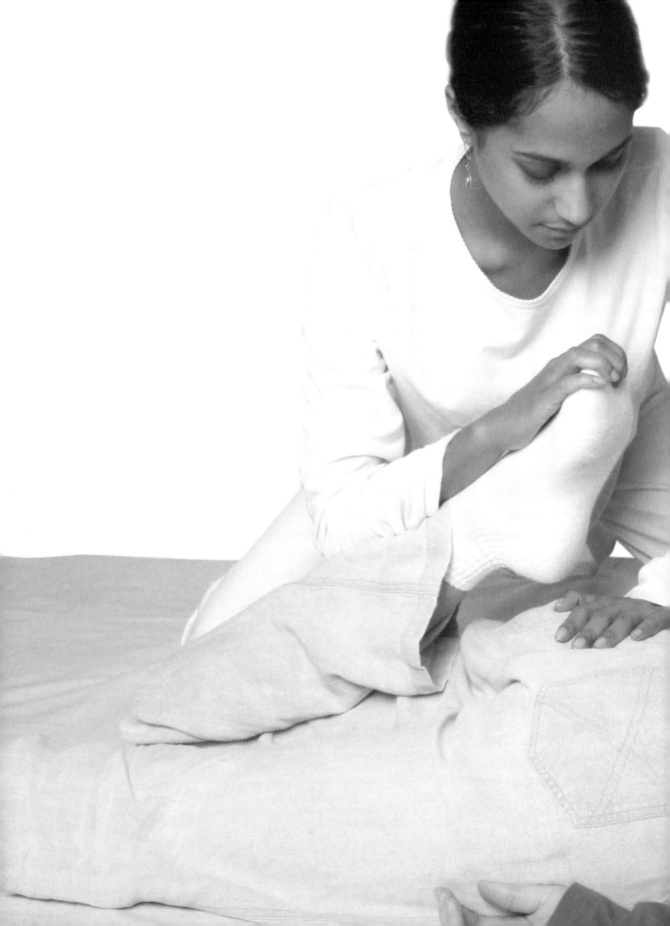

# CHAPTER 4

# Prone Sequence

You are now ready to practise basic technique sequences or 'forms'. If the receiver is new to shiatsu, it is best to start in the prone position, as they will feel less 'exposed' than if they were lying face up or sitting. Make sure he or she is comfortable by placing cushions where necessary.

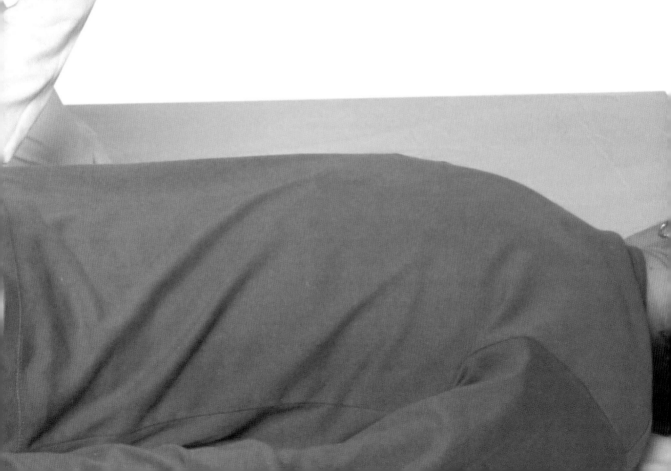

## 4.1 Baby walking

Kneel next to the receiver, ensuring you spread your knees wide enough to give you a low centre of gravity and thus a solid base from which to apply the technique. This position is known as *wide kneeling*. Keep your head up and your hara relaxed and open. Lean forward onto all fours, leaning your body weight through your hands and 'walking' your hands randomly over the receiver's back and buttocks, like a baby crawling. Allow gravity to determine the level of pressure rather than applying pressure through pushing. Relax your hands and allow them to mould into the contours of the receiver's body. Avoid leaning the heel of your hand directly on her spinal column and do not lean too heavily on her lower back. You can extend the technique to the back of the receiver's thighs, but *do not* lean into the back of the knees.

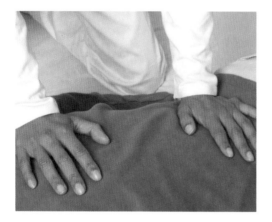

*Relax your hands to allow them to mould into the contours of the receiver's back.*

## 4.2 Palming

Maintain the same stance and posture as in Baby Walking (see opposite). Keep one hand stationary on the side of the receiver's back furthest from you, with the heel of that hand between her spine and shoulder blade. Use your other hand to palm down the back and into the buttock in a line just beyond the far side of the vertebral column. This area of the back relates to the Bladder channel, which in Oriental medicine theory has an influence on the nervous system. This technique will therefore help to calm your receiver in a very direct way.

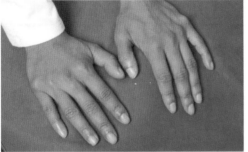

1. Rest one hand between the spine and shoulder blade as you palm down the receiver's back with the other.

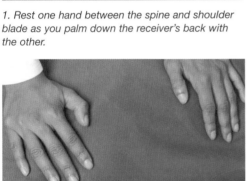

2. Keep the palming hand in a line just beyond the far side of the spine.

3. Palm down the length of the back, towards and into the buttock.

## 4.3 Stretching muscles away from the thoracic spine

This technique is great for relieving stiffness in the upper back. There are two main versions to choose from. Maintain the same stance and posture as in Baby Walking (see page 72). Place both hands on the far side of the receiver's upper back, with the heel of both hands in the natural groove close to her spine. Keep your belly and shoulders relaxed and lean forward, allowing some of your body weight to transfer through your hands into the receiver's back. As with all shiatsu techniques you should never push but where possible let gravity do the work for you.

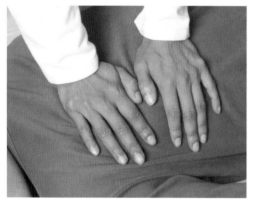

*VERSION A*
*Allow some of your body weight to fall into the receiver's back simultaneously through the heels of both hands, thus stretching the muscles away from the spine. Synchronize your leaning forward with the receiver's exhalations.*

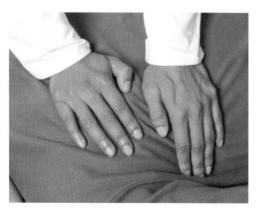

*VERSION B*
*Instead of leaning through both hands simultaneously, shift your weight from one hand to the other so that as the weight increases through one hand it decreases through the other. Do not break contact.*

Note: Do not use this technique in the lower back; the vertebrae of the upper back (thoracic region) are able to rotate along their vertical axis, whereas the vertebrae of the lower back (lumbar region) cannot. Trying to perform this technique in the lower back may strain the ligaments around the vertebrae.

## Moving to the other side

While there are other methods of moving around the receiver, this way is good for developing fluency of movement and hip flexibility. When you have followed the sequence through, you will be ready to repeat the palming technique from the other side of your receiver, having successfully completed a 'transition'.

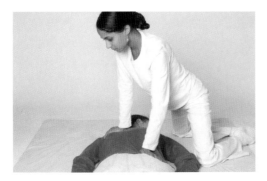

*1. Place one hand on the receiver's nearside lower ribs or buttock. Place your other hand on the far side scapula (shoulder blade).*

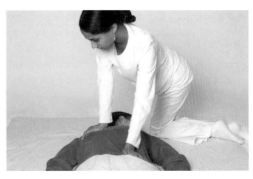

*2. Position your leading knee so there is enough space between your knee and the receiver's nearside shoulder for you to place your trailing knee.*

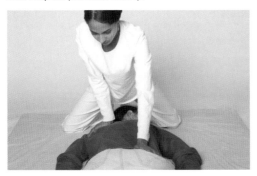

*3. Now move your leading knee to the floor on the other side of the receiver's head, leaving sufficient room for the trailing knee to be placed.*

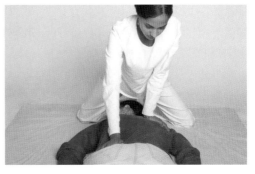

*4. Glide the hand that was on the buttock or lower ribs up to the scapula. Simultaneously, glide the other hand down to the buttock or lower ribs.*

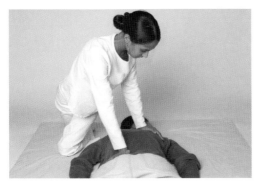

*5. Now move the trailing knee over the receiver's head to rest next to the leading knee.*

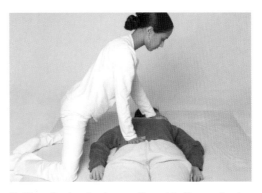

*6. Move the leading knee adjacent to the receiver's waist or hips and make any necessary adjustments to your position for your comfort.*

## 4.4 Rocking

Kneel at right angles to your receiver and place both hands on her torso, on or near her waistline. If preferred, you can place one of your hands on her sacrum or hip. Rock her body from side to side. Attune to the rhythm that seems most natural for her, which you will recognize as the rhythm which is most effortless for you to maintain. Keep your arms, shoulders and spinal column loose and 'soft', allowing the rocking movement to come more from your belly and hips than from your arms. Being rocked is an inherently relaxing experience, as is evidenced by the way that babies are lulled when gently rocked, so this technique is useful to include at this stage if the receiver has not yet fully relaxed.

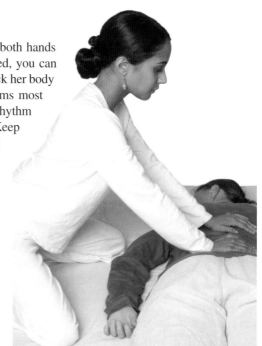

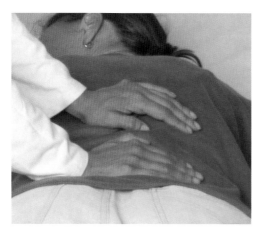

*Mould your hands into the contours of your receiver's waistline, ensuring they are free of tension. 'Connect' rather than grab.*

## 4.5 Diagonal stretch

Place one hand on the near side of the receiver's upper back, with the heel of your hand close to the inside edge of the scapula (shoulder blade) and the palm held flat against the lower half of the scapula. Your hand should be positioned no higher than this otherwise you will compress the receiver's neck. Place your other hand on the receiver's far side buttock so that your hands are positioned diagonally. Lean your hara forward towards the space between your hands and you will feel them tending to splay apart. Allow this splaying effect to take up the slack in the receiver's skin and flesh, thus giving her a diagonal stretch across her entire back. Keep your shoulders down, your belly relaxed and your head up. Move your hands to the opposite scapula and buttock and repeat. Readjust your kneeling position for optimum comfort.

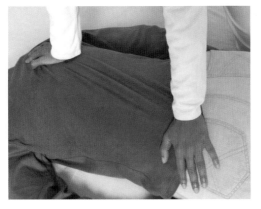

*Place your upper hand partly below and partly over the receiver's shoulder blade. Place your other hand on the opposite buttock. Lean forward, stretching the back diagonally.*

Note: If kneeling on both knees is uncomfortable, try half kneeling with the knee of one leg and the foot of the other on the ground (see page 46).

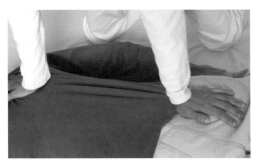

*VARIATION*
*Follow the previous directions but place both hands on the same side of the body. This will 'open' one side of the back at a time in a longitudinal direction rather than diagonally.*

## 4.6 Sacral rub

Adopt whichever kneeling or squatting position suits you. Keep a support hand on the back of the receiver's torso or the back of her thigh. Place your other hand firmly on her sacrum (the bony area between the centre of her buttocks and her lower back). Rotate your hand as if polishing the bony sacrum with the skin covering it, so that the skin and the clothing over it is used like a cleaning rag, for 15–30 seconds. (Do *not* polish her skin or her clothing with the surface of your palm). This technique generates a feeling of deep warmth, which spreads from the sacrum throughout the entire body and is useful for people who tend to feel the cold. If your arms become tired, change hands every five seconds or so.

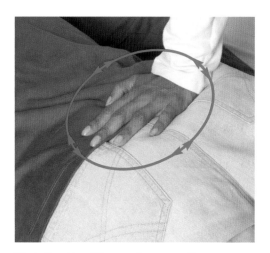

*Circle the skin of the sacral area over the sacral bone.*

## 4.7 Retreating cat

Move from the side of the receiver's body to just beyond her head, facing her feet, using the first half of the procedure described in Moving to the Other Side (see page 75). Glide both hands down her back until the heels of your hands rest into her buttocks. Lean your body weight forward for 1–2 seconds to stretch her buttocks away from her lower back, thus giving a gentle traction to her lower back. Now 'walk' your hands from her buttocks up to her shoulder, removing one hand after the other as if you were crawling backwards away from her lower back. If you like, you can 'walk' your hands into her upper arms. Repeat the Retreating Cat 3–4 times. Glide your hands gracefully into her buttocks; stretching them too suddenly or vigourously away from her lower back could weaken the ligaments of her lumbo-sacral joint and lower lumbar vertebrae.

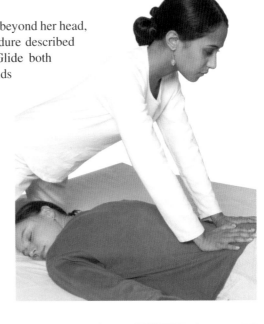

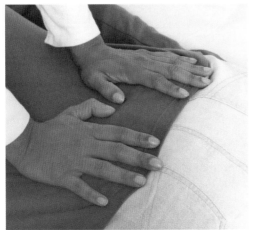

*1. Make sure your hands are well on the buttocks to ensure a gentle traction to the lower back.*

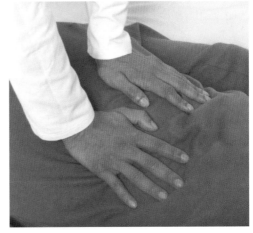

*2. Walk your hands from the buttocks back up to the shoulders.*

## 4.8 Thumbs down Bladder channel on torso

A Ki channel known as the Bladder channel begins in the depression slightly above the inner corner of the eye and runs over the head and down the back about 1½ thumb-widths either side of the vertebral column, all the way into the bony sacrum and down the leg to the foot. This line down the back is known as the *inner line*. Another branch called the *outer line* runs parallel to it at a distance of three thumb-widths from the vertebral column.

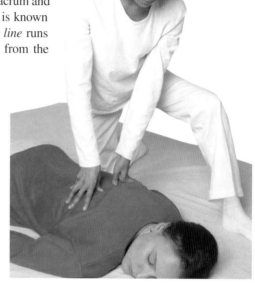

Locate the bony protuberances (the spinous processes) of the vertebral column. Adopt a wide kneeling, half kneeling or squatting position behind the receiver's head. Starting in her upper back, below the base of her neck, glide your thumbs either side of the spine to a position about 1½ thumb-widths lateral to the vertebral column. Lean in with your thumbs so that the angle of pressure is at right angles to the contour of her back. Sink your thumbs in using your body weight, not strength. Check with the receiver that you are not causing her any degree of pain. Withdraw your thumbs and glide them adjacent to the space between the next knobbly spinous processes. Continue working down the receiver's back in this manner until you reach a stage where it is no longer possible for you to keep your hara in line with the neck of the tsubo that you are working on.

To maintain the correct angle of entry into the tsubos of the Bladder channel, change your position by moving away from the receiver's head and adopting a half-kneeling position by her side, facing towards her head. Work down her lower thoracic region into the lumbar area, if necessary shuffling your position slightly as you move down to make yourself comfortable. As you work towards and onto the sacrum (buttock area) you may prefer to turn and face the receiver's feet in order to ensure the correct angle of entry into the tsubo.

Go back to the head of the receiver's body, facing her feet, trying not to take your hand off her body as you do so. Repeat, but this time, work three thumb-widths from the midline of the vertebral column.

Where the Bladder channel runs along the spine it has points, which relate to different organs and functions of the body. Experienced practitioners may focus on these points (tsubos) in order to alleviate specific problems, but at beginner's level it is sufficient for you to know that by working down the Bladder channel in a generalized way as described in this technique you will be encouraging greater harmony between all the receiver's bodily functions.

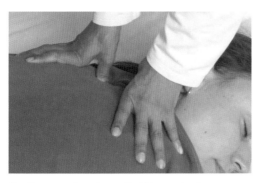

Position your thumbs so that the angle of pressure is at right angles to the contour of the back.

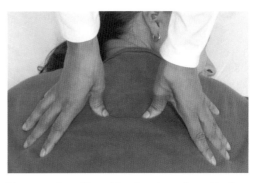

The correct position of the thumbs, adjacent to the space between the spinous processes.

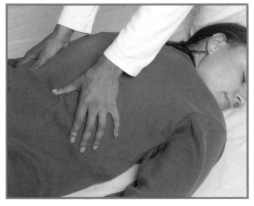

STOP  The thumbs are too far down the receiver's back in relation to the giver's position, so that the giver's hara is no longer aligned with the neck of the tsubo.

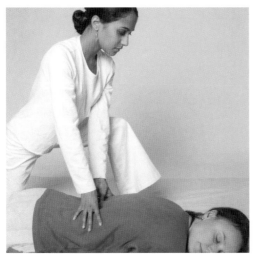

1. In half kneeling, facing towards her head, work down the lower thoracic area of the Bladder channel, either side of the spine.

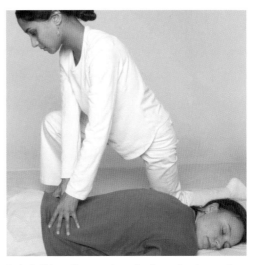

2. In half kneeling, work on the lower lumbar and sacral area, facing towards the receiver's feet if you prefer.

## 4.9 Palm/forearm down back of legs

Kneel or half kneel beside the receiver with one knee or foot adjacent to her hip and the other adjacent to her knee or lower leg. Place your support hand on her sacrum or nearside buttock and use the other hand to palm down the back of her thigh as far as the back of the knee. Do not lean pressure into the back of her knee, although you can make a light connection there with your palm.

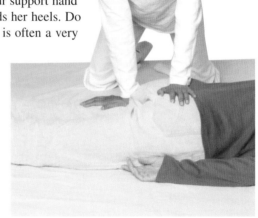

Move your position closer to her feet so that your support hand now rests on her lower thigh. Palm down towards her heels. Do not lean excessive pressure into her calf, as this is often a very sensitive area.

Without breaking contact, move back up so that your knee is again adjacent to her hip. This time rest a hand or forearm against her buttock for support and use your other forearm to lean pressure into the back of her thigh. Do not look down, but feel your way.

Finally, move your position closer to her feet so that you can again rest a support hand on her lower thigh, and repeat palming your hand towards her heels.

The back of the legs relates predominantly to the Bladder channel, so working this area immediately after using your thumbs down the Bladder channel in the torso will give the receiver a better sense of 'connectedness' between her torso and her legs.

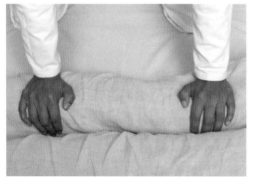

*1. Rest your support hand on the lower thigh as your other hand palms down towards the feet.*

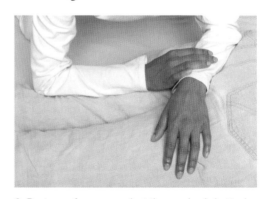

*2. Rest your forearm against the receiver's buttock for support and use your other forearm to lean pressure into the back of her thigh.*

Note: Avoid the legs if varicose veins are present because direct pressure on varicose veins is extremely painful and may cause them damage.

## 4.10 Heel to buttock

With one knee adjacent to the receiver's hip and the other approximately adjacent to her knee, place your support hand on her buttock and your other hand under her instep. Keeping your chest within 12 inches (30 cm) of her foot, bring her heel towards her buttock, at the same time using your support hand to stretch her buttock away from her lower back. The movement should be performed in a slightly circular rather than linear manner so that you bring the heel towards the buttock along a semi-circular path and draw it back in a similar fashion.

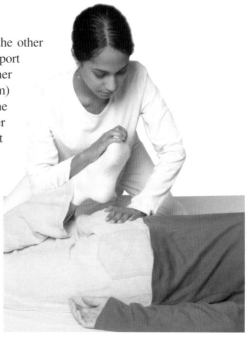

If the receiver's heel does not easily reach her buttock, recognize the point of resistance and do not force the stretch. If the receiver is so flexible that she feels no stretch in the thigh muscles with this technique, you can increase the stretch by raising her thigh upon your own before leaning her heel towards her buttock.

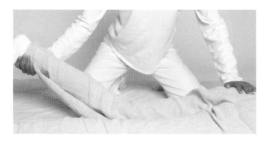

*1. The starting position: the support hand is on the buttock and the other hand is under the instep.*

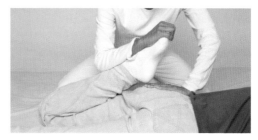

*2. Bring her heel towards her buttock, simultaneously stretching her buttock away from her lower back with your support hand.*

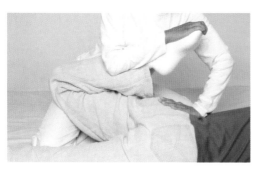

*3. To increase the stretch for flexible recipients, raise her knee onto your thigh prior to applying the stretch.*

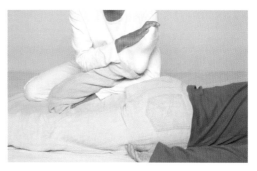

*VARIATION*
*This variation gives less stretch to the front of the thigh but 'opens' the front of the knee joint by way of slight leverage. Because your hand is sandwiched behind the knee, the front of the knee is stretched open a little.*

## 4.11 Forearms into soles

When you bring the receiver's leg down out of the Heel to Buttock technique, position your thigh so that her instep comes to rest upon it. The concave shape of her instep should fit precisely into the convex contour of your thigh, so that her foot is fully supported and not dangling in mid-air. Your other knee should rest on the back of her thigh, although if this is difficult you can rest it on the floor. Lean your forearm into the sole of her foot, keeping your wrist fully relaxed.

Because the soles of the feet are our main connecting points to the earth, leaning good solid pressure into them will give a sense of groundedness, particularly for those who are rather fuzzyheaded. Apart from that, this technique also feels very pleasant to receive. However, as some people have extremely sensitive feet, ask your receiver if she is actually enjoying it and if not, stop!

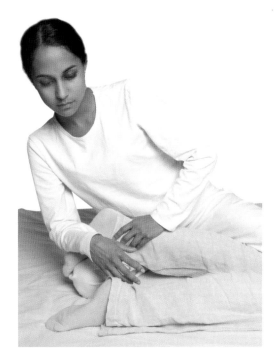

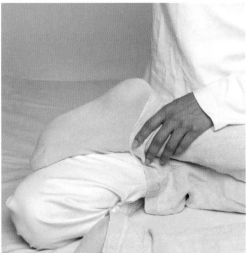

*Make sure the receiver's instep moulds precisely into the contour of your thigh to give full support to her foot.*

## Moving to the other side

This sequence shows you how to get to the other side of the receiver's body smoothly and without breaking contact. Upon completion of this manoeuvre you will be in the correct position to repeat the entire leg sequence from 4.9 to 4.11 from the other side of the receiver.

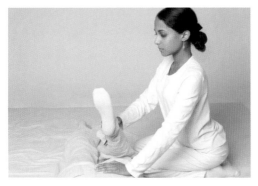

*1. Bring her heel towards her buttock. Position your leading knee so that there is enough space between your knee and her nearside knee for you to place your trailing knee.*

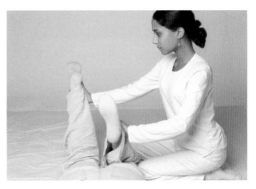

*2. Adjust your hands so that the hand that was on the buttock now holds the nearside foot. Use your other hand to raise her other foot from the ground.*

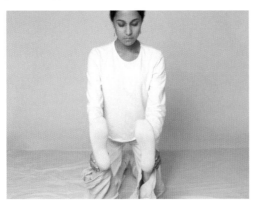

*3. Now move your leading knee to the floor beyond her far side knee, leaving sufficient room for the trailing knee to be placed.*

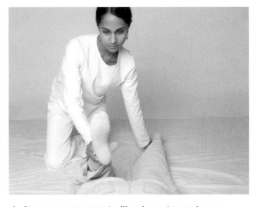

*4. As you move your trailing knee towards your leading knee, lower her far side foot to the ground.*

*5. Now position your hands and adjust your leg position as if to perform the Heel to Buttock stretch on this side.*

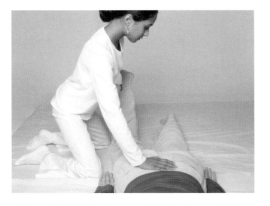

Repeat the techniques 4.9 to 4.11 from the other side of the receiver.

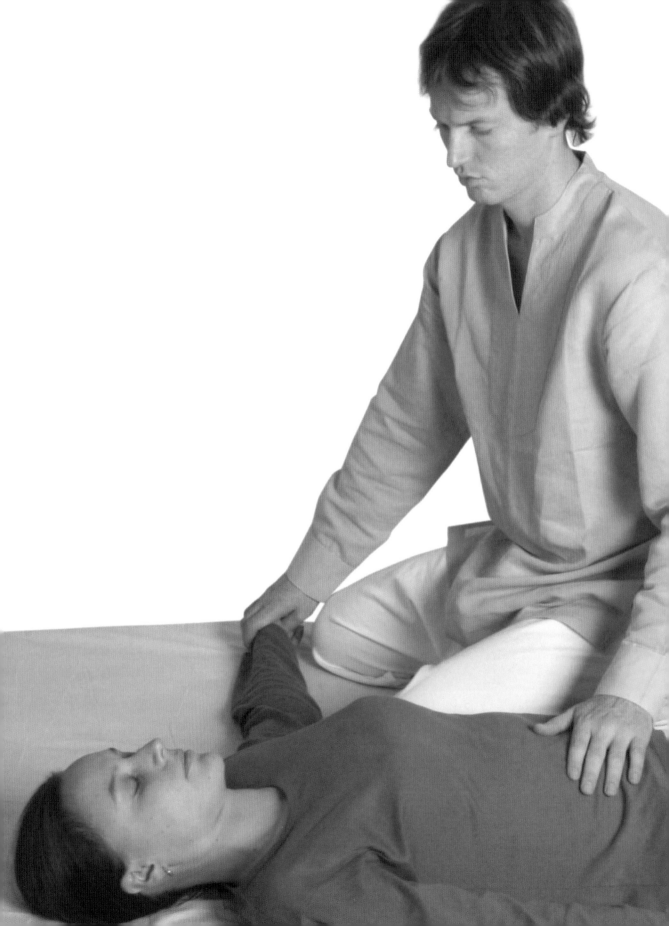

# CHAPTER 5

# Supine Sequence

When giving shiatsu in this position, ask your receiver if she would like a pillow under her head. If she is very round-shouldered her chin will protrude upwards, constricting the back of her neck and overstretching the front, and she will be more comfortable with a block of 1–2 inches (2.5–5 cm) thickness beneath her head. A book or a very stiff cushion will suffice. Before you begin, try to reach an attunement with the receiver by spending about a minute kneeling by her with one hand resting on her hara and your other hand holding her wrist or hand, as shown here.

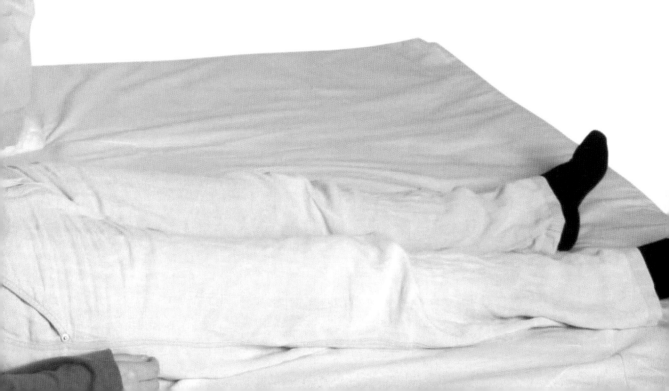

## 5.1 Pulling heels

This technique gently stretches the recipient's spine. Stand at the receiver's feet, facing towards her head. Place your hands under her heels and pick up her feet. Ensure her heels are lifted high enough for her lower back to flatten against the floor; otherwise you may exaggerate your own lumbar curve. Do not clutch her ankles; hold onto the bony part of her heels. Adopt a stance with your knees slightly bent and your feet slightly apart and hold her feet close to your belly or chest.

If the receiver has hyper-extended knee joints (knees which seem to bend the other way slightly when the leg is meant to be straight) as well as heavy legs, avoid this technique.

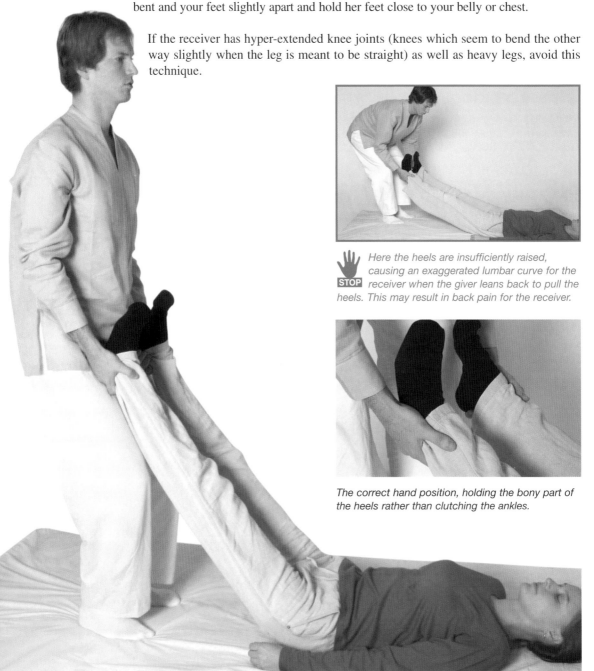

**STOP** *Here the heels are insufficiently raised, causing an exaggerated lumbar curve for the receiver when the giver leans back to pull the heels. This may result in back pain for the receiver.*

*The correct hand position, holding the bony part of the heels rather than clutching the ankles.*

## 5.2 Double knee to chest

Still holding the receiver's heels, walk forwards as you raise her heels level with your chest. You may want to rest her heels on your chest for a moment as you put your hands behind her knees. Allow her knees to bend as you walk your feet adjacent to her hips, using the inside surface of your knees or lower legs to support and control her legs. Gently lean some of your weight through your hands straight down onto her legs, allowing her knees to spread to avoid pressure on her aorta (the main blood vessel from the heart). This will give a subtle 'opening' stretch to her lower back and buttocks and will help decongest her colon. To move out of this technique, see below.

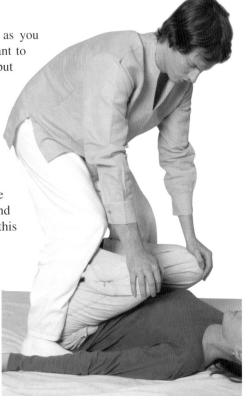

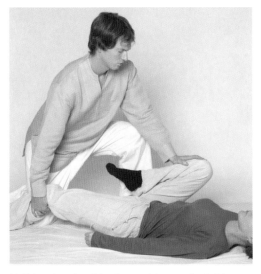

*Half-kneel to the side of one of the receiver's hips and lower her legs to the ground, one at a time. Ensure you support the back of her knee as you do so. This option works better on the smaller, lighter receiver.*

## 5.3 Hip circling

There are several versions of Hip Circling. The three most popular options are given here. All involve bending one of the receiver's legs towards her chest and drawing outward circles in the air with her knee. The Hip Circling technique gently mobilizes the hip joints and increases circulation to the hips and sacrum.

Hip Circling illustrates how truly relaxed your receiver is because unless she is fully at ease she will hold tension in her leg throughout the movement, often doing the movement herself instead of allowing you to do it. If this is the case Version B should work better because the extra support will make it easier for her to let go. Give her plenty of time and encouragement so that she feels able to 'give' her leg to you.

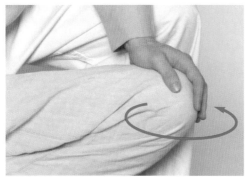

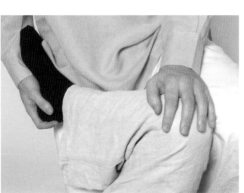

*VERSION A*
*Adopt the half-kneeling position to one side of the receiver's hip. Hold her knee with one hand and her heel with the other. Bend her knee towards her chest. Draw outward circles in the air with her leg, exploring the natural range of movement in her hip joint. This method allows for the maximum circumference of hip rotation. Alternatively, you can keep your leg in contact with her moving leg instead, which restricts the range of movement but adds a greater sense of 'connection'.*

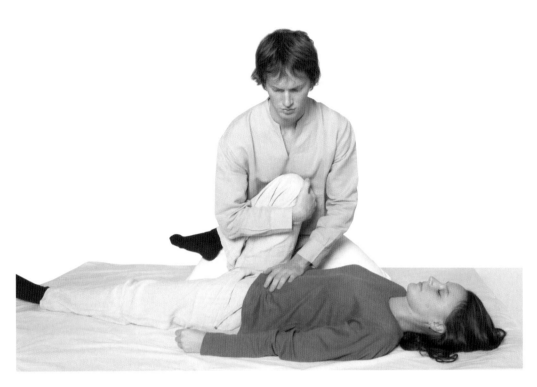

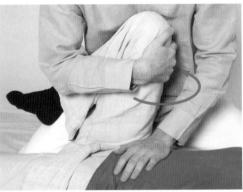

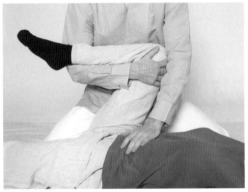

*VERSION B*
*Adopt the wide kneeling position. Place one hand on the receiver's belly. Hold her knee with your other hand, hugging her folded leg between your chest and forearm. Rotate her hip joint by circling your torso from your hara, thereby circling her leg. This method does not allow full circumference of hip rotation, but gives a much greater sense of nurturing and connection.*

*VERSION C*
*This version of Hip Circling is the same as Version B, except that your forearm cradles the receiver's lower leg. Some receivers may find this version rather too intimate and consequently fail to relax into it. This technique may also be done in the squat kneeling position if you find it more comfortable.*

## 5.4 Single knee to chest

Either version of Hip Circling can be progressed into the Single Knee to Chest technique by simply leaning some of your weight towards the receiver's chest, keeping one hand on either her belly, or the straight leg. This can be helpful if that leg has a tendency to lift up as you lean some of your weight onto the bent leg. On some people the knee will more naturally move to the side of their torso; on others, the knee will move directly towards the chest. Go with her natural direction. The technique will stretch the lower back and buttocks and help to decongest the colon.

Do this technique slowly so that you go no further than is comfortable for the receiver. If she does begin to feel discomfort her back and neck may stiffen, causing her chin to protrude.

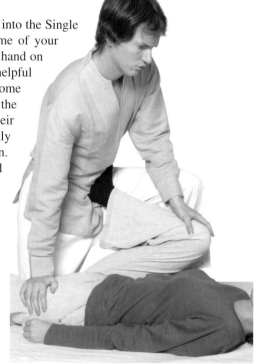

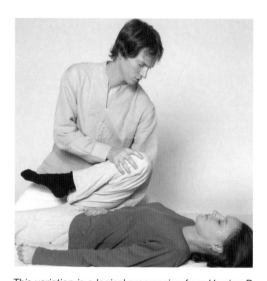

*This variation is a logical progression from Version B of Hip Circling. Adopt wide kneeling or squat kneeling (see pages 46–47) and keep one hand on the receiver's belly as you apply gentle pressure onto the bent knee.*

## 5.5 Stretch outside of thigh

This stretch 'opens' the channel relating to the Gallbladder. Place the receiver's foot on the floor next to the knee of her straight leg, with her knee pointing towards the ceiling. Place one hand on her knee and your other hand firmly on her hip to anchor it. Place your foot or knee (depending on whether you are half-kneeling or kneeling) against her foot to prevent it from slipping. Then give a slow stretch to the lateral side of her thigh by leaning her knee away from you. Sometimes it works better if the foot of the receiver's bent leg is placed across her straight leg, with her foot against the outside of her straight leg knee.

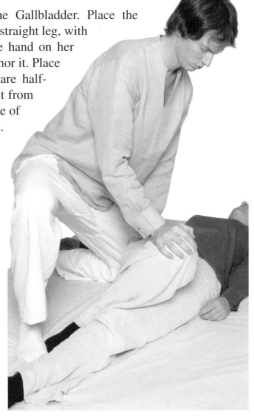

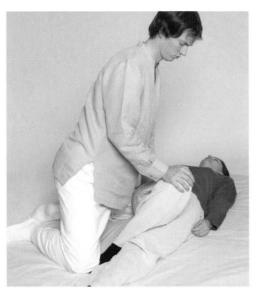

*In the kneeling position, the giver's knee anchors the receiver's foot to prevent it sliding away.*

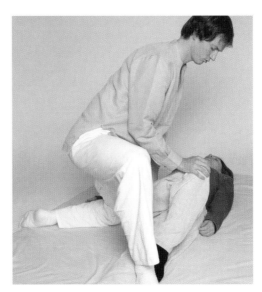

*VARIATION*
*The receiver's bent leg can be placed across her straight leg.*

## 5.6 Opening inside leg and pelvis

Keeping the receiver's leg in the same starting position as the previous technique, adjust your legs to the opposite half-kneeling position. Place a cushion or two on the floor where her knee will rest when you lower her knee outwards towards the ground. As you lower her knee, switch your hand position so that the hand that was on the hip now supports the knee and the hand that was on the knee moves to anchor the upper thigh/hip of the far side leg. Gently 'open' her pelvis and inner thigh muscles by leaning the knee gently into the supporting cushions. Do not look down, but let your hara relax down. You may need more cushions, depending on the receiver's flexibility. If you do not have cushions nearby, allow her knee to be supported by your lower leg or inner ankle.

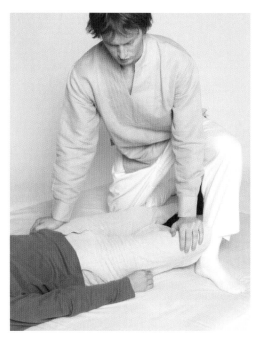

*If no cushion is available, the receiver's knee can be supported by the giver's lower leg.*

## 5.7 Foot to hara

Support the receiver's leg as you straighten it and position yourself in wide kneeling so that the outside edge of her foot rests squarely in your hara, embraced by your two hands. Lean your hara into her foot and circle her foot using your whole body. If the receiver has hyper-extended knees (knees that bend the wrong way slightly) or experiences discomfort in her knee during this technique, use one hand or some cushions to support the back of her knee, thus keeping her knee 'unlocked'.

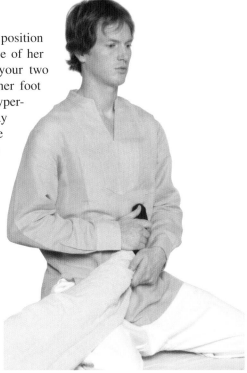

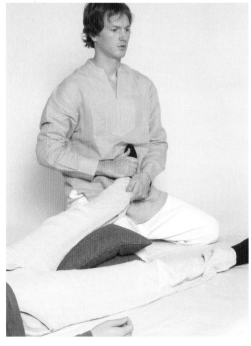

*Provide support beneath the knee by means of a cushion if the receiver has hyper-extended knees or is experiencing discomfort.*

Repeat techniques 3–7 on the other leg, trying not to break contact as you take your time moving across.

## 5.8 Arm circling and palming down arm

Move from the receiver's foot to her arm slowly and carefully, trying to maintain hand-to-body contact throughout. Cup one hand on the receiver's upper chest and shoulder and the other hand close by on her upper arm. Lean down with fairly firm supportive pressure for about 10 seconds. This will encourage her shoulder joint to 'let go'. Now move your hand from her upper arm to her wrist, with your thumb held against the palm of her hand. Take a step back with your outside leg and bring her hand to your own shoulder, simultaneously adjusting the hand which is on her shoulder to ensure sufficient purchase to stretch her shoulder. Take a big step forward with your outside leg to stretch her arm beyond her head. Step forwards and backwards two or three times to rotate the shoulder joint. The receiver's arm should be taken forward through a vertical arc and brought back

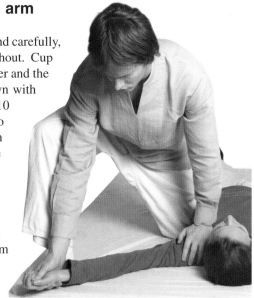

through a horizontal arc close to the floor. You should maintain some traction to the shoulder joint throughout, particularly when you take the arm upwards and forwards.

Now place her arm on the floor at right angles to her torso. Palm down her arm towards her wrist, keeping one foot on her palm if you can remain comfortable like that as this will create an extra connection. If not, place your foot somewhere on the ground that feels more comfortable. Try to keep your other leg in contact with the side of her body to give maximum connection. If her arms are very long in relation to your size, place her arm closer to her body and, if necessary, sacrifice the connection of your leg against her torso.

Arm Circling mobilizes the shoulder joint, increasing the circulation of Ki and blood to the shoulder and chest area.

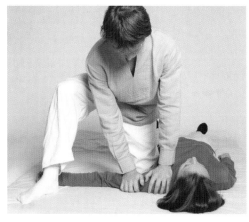

*1. Place one hand on the receiver's upper chest and shoulder and the other hand on her upper arm.*

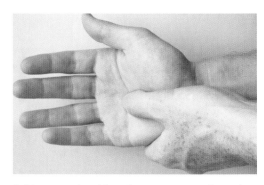

*2. Move your hand from her upper arm to her wrist and place your thumb against her palm.*

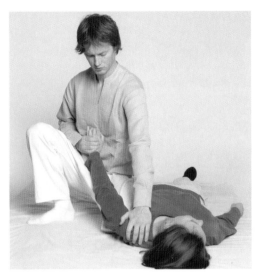

3. Stepping back with your outside leg results in a stretch to the recipient's trapezius muscle.

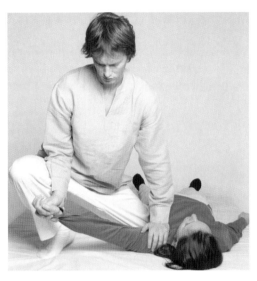

4. A big step forwards allows you to stretch the receiver's arm up beyond her head.

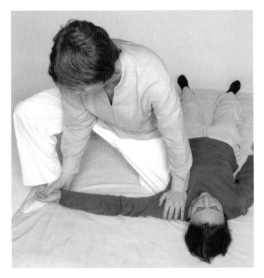

5. Repeat Arm Circling two or three times, bringing the arm back in a horizontal arc close to the ground.

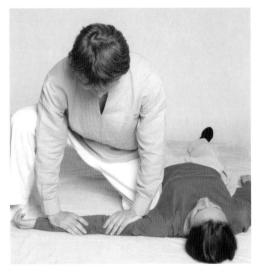

6. Lay the receiver's arm on the ground at right angles to her torso and palm down her arm towards her wrist.

Note: Rotate the receiver's arm overhead only as far as she can go before her shoulder tightens up – do not take the arm to the floor if it will not easily go there. This is likely to be the case if your receiver is round-shouldered.

## Moving to the other side via the head

There are several ways to get from one side of the receiver's body to the other without taking both your hands off her body. The method shown here works particularly well if you are taller than the receiver. If you are shorter, just take a few extra shuffles with your knees as you go.

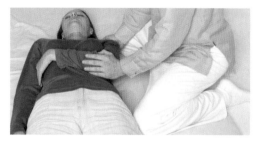

*1. Kneeling with your knees well spread, place the receiver's forearm across her lower ribs, holding her elbow and shoulder.*

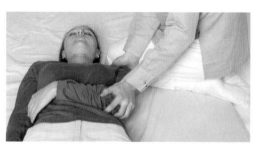

*2. Make sure there is space between your leading knee and her shoulder. Place your trailing knee next to your leading knee.*

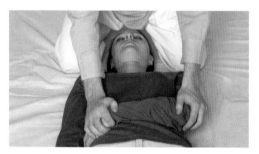

*3. Move your leading knee to the floor on the other side of her head, making sure you leave space between your knee and her head. Simultaneously move your hand from her shoulder to her wrist.*

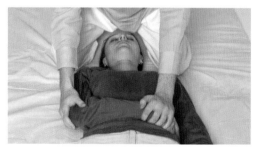

*4. Place her arm back on the floor and bring her other forearm across her lower ribs.*

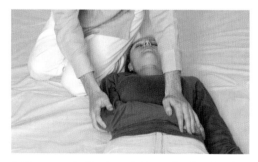

*5. Place your trailing knee between her head and your leading knee.*

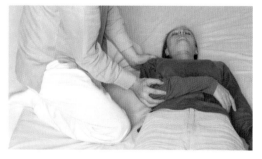

*6. Move your leading knee near to her hip, at the same time moving your hand from her wrist to her shoulder.*

Repeat Arm Circling and Palming Down Arm from the other side on the arm you are now holding.

## 5.9 Shoulder press

Position yourself at the receiver's head, looking towards her feet. Check to see if she has round shoulders. If so, her shoulders will not lie flat upon the ground and her chin will project upwards. If this is the case, or if she has neck pain, follow the variation shown below right. Otherwise proceed as follows: cup your hands over her shoulders, fingers to the rear. The heels of your hands should be on the upper chest muscles (pectoralis minor), in the hollow just below her clavicle (collarbone). Lean your hara forward so that your weight falls through your hands, 'opening' the receiver's upper chest. Be careful to keep your groin well away from her face, and tuck away any loose, dangling clothing to prevent it contacting her head.

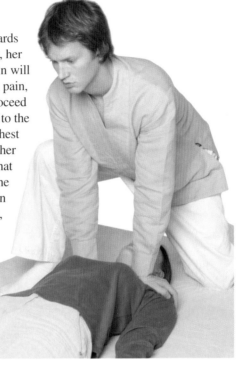

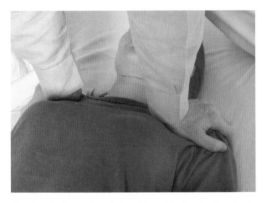

*The heel of your hand should rest in the hollow just below the collarbone and your fingers should be to the rear.*

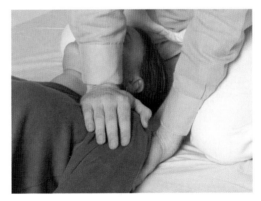

*VARIATION*
*For those receivers who have round shoulders or neck pain or who are frail, place one hand underneath the shoulder to support it and place the other hand on the upper chest and shoulder, thereby sandwiching the shoulder between your hands. Lean through your upper hand. Repeat on the other shoulder.*

## 5.10 Hand to hara

This technique calms the Heart channel and consequently calms the mind. Adopt the wide kneeling position. Bring one of the receiver's arms onto your thigh and hold the back of her hand against your hara. If you have her right hand in your hara, hold it with your left hand and vice versa. Rest your other hand on her armpit or upper arm, and then slowly lean gentle pressure through your hand along her arm towards her elbow. Alternatively, a mild squeezing or stroking action can be applied. Sometimes it works better to lean your forearm in rather than use your hand; especially when working down their forearm.

To complete the technique, use two or three fingers of your other hand to apply gentle pressure to the anterior surface of the receiver's wrist, in line with her fifth finger. Repeat on her other arm. Replace her arm on the ground by her side to conclude.

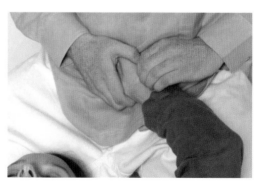

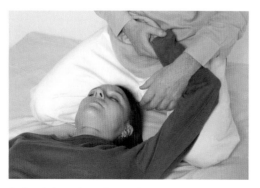

1. Support the receiver's arm on your thigh and hold her hand against your hara. Then palm along the upper arm towards the elbow.

3. Finally, use two or three fingers to apply gentle pressure to the anterior surface of her wrist, in line with her fifth finger.

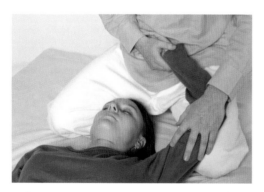

2. Gently lean through your forearm along the receiver's forearm.

## 5.11 Fingertips into suboccipital area

Cradle the receiver's head in your hands and rest the back of your hands on the floor. Move your knees back far enough to rest your elbows on the floor and to allow your back, hara and chest to remain open and relaxed. Rest your fingertips into the area of the receiver's neck closest to the back of her skull (the occiput). By lightly flexing your wrists you can tilt her head back a little, allowing greater depth of contact with your fingertips.

To conclude this technique, and the supine sequence, gently withdraw your hands via the back of her head extremely slowly, thus giving a very mild lengthening effect to the back of her neck.

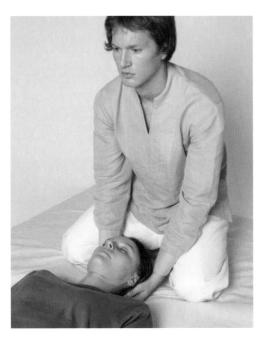

*VARIATION*
*Some practitioners find it more comfortable to be positioned closer, sitting up. Others find that this method closes the hara too much. Try both positions to see which suits you best.*

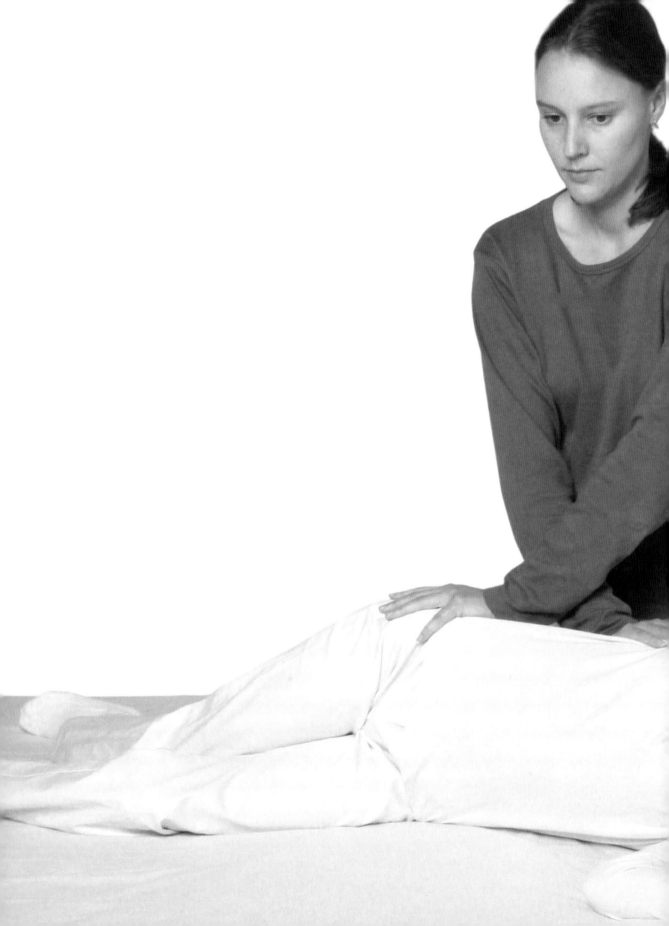

# CHAPTER 6
# Side Sequence

Shiatsu in the side position has certain advantages over shiatsu in the prone or supine position, as it enables full mobility of the shoulders, arms, hips and legs, plus greater movement of the torso. Also, persons with back problems, or women in the later stages of pregnancy often find it difficult to fully relax in any position other than the side position.

To ensure the receiver is comfortable in the side position, place sufficient padding under their head and knee, as shown on page 106.

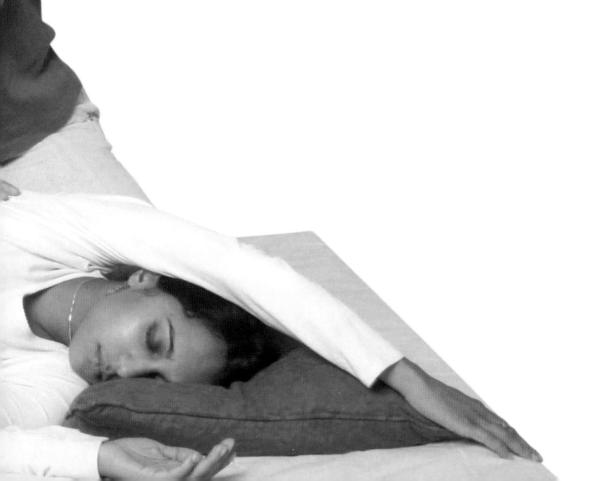

## 6.1 Trapezius stretch

Kneel in the seiza position next to the receiver, facing towards her head. Snuggle in close for maximum connection, but without pushing her off balance. Place her forearm over your forearm so that her arm does not drag on the floor. Clasping your hands around her shoulder, lean back, using your body weight to 'open' her neck (upper trapezius muscle). If her head comes away from the pillow you have leaned back far too strongly, so go more gently. Your hand position can be such that one hand overlaps the other, as shown here, or you can interlace your fingers. Do what you find most comfortable.

The Trapezius Stretch is a great antidote to the stress-induced tension that can so easily accumulate in the neck and shoulders.

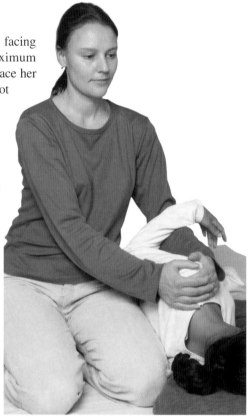

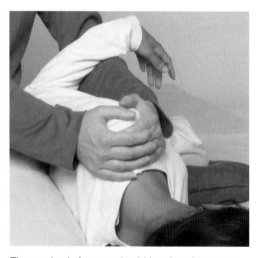

*The receiver's forearm should be placed over your forearm to prevent her arm dragging on the floor.*

## 6.2 Shoulder girdle rotation

From the Trapezius Stretch, rotate the receiver's shoulder girdle in an up, back and down direction to encourage her chest to 'open'. Your whole body should be involved in the rotation, not just your arms. Alternate between the Trapezius Stretch and Shoulder Girdle Rotation for 1–2 minutes.

During this technique some receivers will involuntarily stiffen their shoulder as you try to rotate it. They will tend to relax more if you support the shoulder solidly between your hands. Receivers who are able to relax fully find this technique very pleasant.

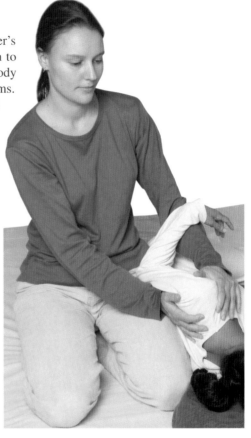

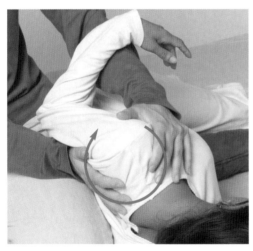

*Correct technique: backward rotations encourage the chest to 'open'.*

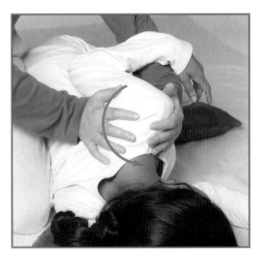

 *Incorrect technique: forward rotations encourage the chest to 'close'.*

## 6.3 Vertical arm stretch

From Shoulder Girdle Rotation, remove your hand from behind the receiver's shoulder and clasp her hand. Leave your other hand on her shoulder and swivel up into half kneeling to face the same direction as she is facing. Sink down a little and embrace her arm, giving it as much contact as possible with your arm and torso. Straighten your posture. This will result in a traction of her shoulder girdle, shoulder, elbow and wrist joints.

Do not be tempted to hold her wrist with both hands, as this may cause undue strain to her wrist or elbow joints. Do not perform this technique from the high kneeling position because that will cause unnecessary stress to your lower back, especially if you have any history of weakness or injury to your back.

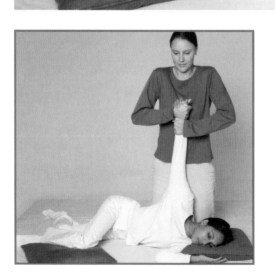

*Incorrect technique: keeping both knees on the ground will cause stress to your lower back. Holding the receiver's wrist without supporting the rest of her arm will stress her shoulder, elbow and wrist joints and cause tension in your neck and shoulders.*

## 6.4 Lance stretch

From the Vertical Arm Stretch, change your grip to hold the receiver's wrist and circle her arm to a position where her arm is projecting beyond her head, so that there is a straight line between her upper hip, shoulder and hand. The hand that was holding her shoulder is now clasped around her upper arm. Rest your forearm upon your knee and lean away from the receiver's feet. This will 'open' the side of her ribs and torso. If her shoulder is stiff, stretch her arm slightly forward.

For this technique, it is best for your receiver to be wearing a long-sleeved garment as otherwise you could overstretch the skin of her upper arm. If she is wearing short sleeves, put a cloth between your hand and her arm.

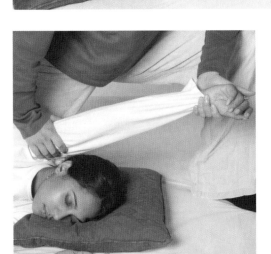

Hold the receiver's wrist and upper arm. Lean away from her feet to stretch her shoulder and 'open' the side of her ribs and torso.

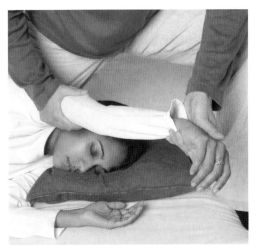

Stretch her arm slightly forward if her shoulder is stiff.

## 6.5 Bent arm lance stretch

Adjust your right foot, placing it well forward of the receiver's head. Allow her arm to bend over your thigh. Clasp her upper arm and hold her forearm. Now, just as in the straight arm Lance Stretch, lean away from her feet. This technique will 'open' the armpit area more than the Straight Arm Lance Stretch.

If you prefer, you can perform the technique in the squat kneeling position. This variation generally works better if your receiver has short arms or you have long legs.

The Bent Arm Lance Stretch helps to expand the rib cage and thus facilitates the ability to breathe more deeply.

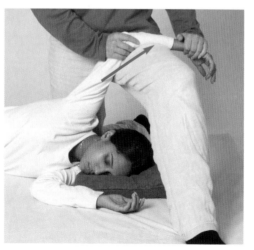

*Place your foot well forward of the receiver's head so that your thigh can support her arm.*

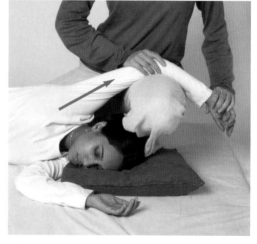

*VARIATION*
*You can also perform this technique in a squat kneeling position. Experiment to see which method is most comfortable for you.*

## 6.6 Side torso gallbladder stretch

Place the receiver's hand on the floor beyond her head or, if her shoulder joint lacks full mobility, in front of her chest. Kneel or half kneel behind her midway between her hip and shoulder. Place her upper leg to rest just behind her lower leg. This allows a greater stretch at the waist. If this is not comfortable for her, leave the leg where it was. Cross your arms and place one hand on her hip and the other hand on her lower ribs. Lean down and 'open' her waist area. Make sure you do not lean into her armpit or shoulder area, as this will cause pain in her neck and shoulder.

This stretch gives the receiver a tremendous sense of 'freeing up' around the waist, lower back and belly. Using the forearms, as in the variation shown right, adds a more supportive, nurturing quality.

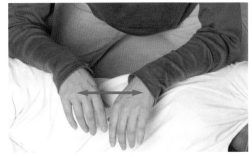

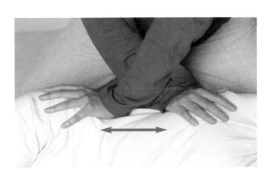

*Leaning through crossed arms effectively 'opens' the waist area.*

*VARIATION*
*Try using your forearms instead of your hands. Again, avoid leaning too close to her armpit.*

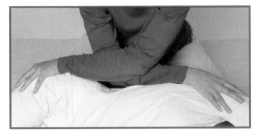

 *Incorrect technique: leaning into the receiver's armpit or shoulder will cause pain in her neck and shoulder.*

## 6.7 Arm to body stretch

Place the receiver's arm along her side with a cushion between her arm and her waist to avoid stressing her elbow joint. Lean your palms into varying areas along her arm and wrist. Do not lean too strongly into the corner of her shoulder as this may cause discomfort to her neck.

This technique is a good counter-movement to techniques 6.3, 6.4, 6.5, and 6.6. It also increases blood and Ki circulation throughout the arm and shoulder.

The forearm variation shown below adds a more warming, supportive quality. Take care not to push the receiver forward as you lean down.

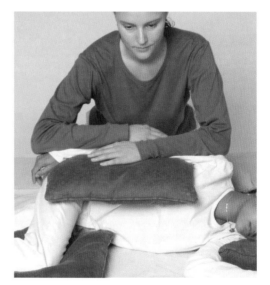

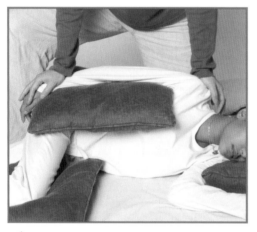

*Incorrect technique: placing your hand too close to the corner of the receiver's shoulder may cause discomfort to her neck.*

*VARIATON*
*Try using your forearms instead of your hands. Again, avoid leaning too close to the receiver's armpit.*

## 6.8 Shoulder girdle dispersing

Kneel or squat kneel next to the receiver, facing towards her head. Snuggle in close for maximum connection, but without pushing her off balance. Place her forearm over your forearm so that her arm does not drag on the floor. Support and anchor her shoulder with one hand while you vigorously circle the heel of your other hand into and around her scapula (shoulder blade). Try to involve your torso in the movement as much as possible so that you minimize tension in your arm. However, your arm will still work quite hard in this technique. You can also try circling your hand slowly and deeply as a variation.

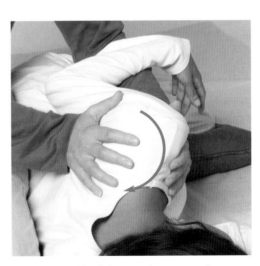

The purpose of this technique is to disperse tension in the muscles between the scapula and the vertebral column, so that the following technique (Sub-scapula Loosening) can be achieved.

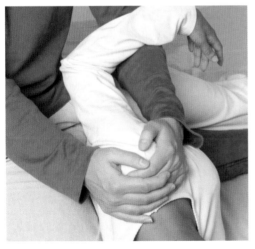

*1. Place the receiver's forearm over your forearm to prevent her arm dragging on the floor.*

*2. Circle the skin of the scapula area over the scapula bone.*

## 6.9 Sub-scapula loosening

Still supporting and anchoring her shoulder, place the receiver's hand behind her back. Place your fingertips under the inside edge of her scapula (shoulder blade) with your forearm resting on your thigh to anchor it, so that it becomes a fulcrum. Fold the receiver's scapula over your fingertips, and lean away from her body, levering the scapula away from her rib cage a little. This looks extremely uncomfortable, but very few receivers feel any sensation at all during this technique, which is nicknamed 'the chicken wing'.

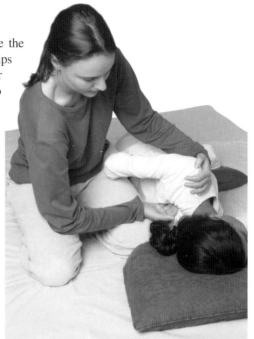

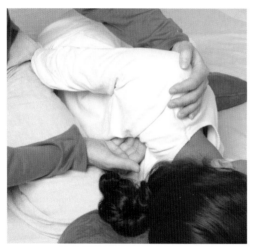

1. Position the receiver's arm behind her back to make it easier to get your fingers beneath her scapula. Rest your forearm on your thigh to anchor it, thus reducing the need to tense your arm.

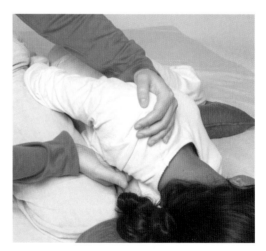

2. As you lean away the scapula is pulled away from the rib cage, releasing trapped Ki from that area.

Notes: You may find that you cannot get your fingers under the scapula. If so, try various alterations to the receiver's arm position. If you still cannot get your fingers in, give up. Some scapulae are simply too small or too tight against the ribs. When one scapula is very mobile and easy to get underneath and the other is too tight, this often indicates a postural anomaly such as scoliosis (twisted spine). If the stiff scapula is on the right it can also be a sign of a congested liver. Pain under the left scapula may indicate certain stomach problems such as stomach ulcer or chronic indigestion.

## 6.10 Head press

Come up into half kneeling or squat kneeling, facing towards the receiver's head. Place both palms on her head, being careful not to cover her ears. (You may wish to place a cloth between her head and your hands, especially if her hair is greasy). Lean forward so that your weight drops through your hands – the pressure should obviously be gentle. Try to distribute your weight evenly throughout the palms of your hands rather than focusing it into the heels of your hands.

The channel relating to the gallbladder covers much of the side of the head and there are many points (tsubos) on this part of the channel that alleviate pain in the head, ears and eyes. This technique can therefore have a beneficial effect upon those symptoms. Note, however, that too much pressure will have the opposite effect.

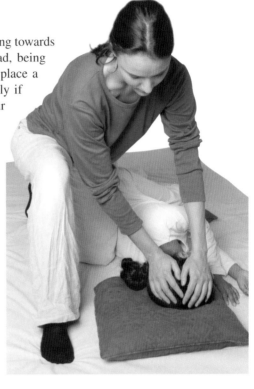

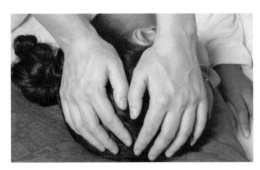

*1. Place your hands on the receiver's head in such a way that you do not cover her ears.*

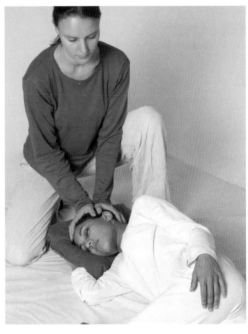

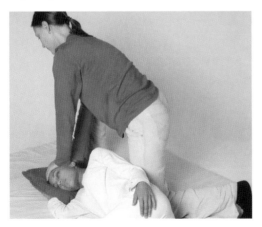

*2. Lean forward so that you use your weight rather than your strength to apply pressure.*

*VARIATION*
*Adopt the same stances, but apply the technique from a position beyond the receiver's head, facing towards her feet.*

## 6.11 Occipital opening/neck release

Squat kneel beside the receiver. Snuggle in close for maximum connection, but without pushing her off balance. Place one hand on her forehead, without obstructing her eyes. Ideally, connect the front of her shoulder with your forearm (if it compromises your comfort, abandon this connection). Place the heel of your other hand against the nape of her neck and occiput. Explore this area with mild pressure.

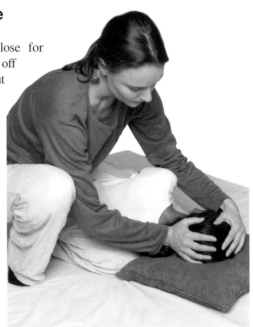

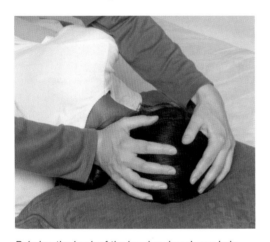

*Palming the back of the head and neck can help relieve eye fatigue or a mild headache.*

## 6.12 Knees into back

Squat behind the receiver with one hand on her shoulder and your other hand on her hip. Lean your knees against her back above her spinal column, upon the Bladder channel found $1\frac{1}{2}$ thumb-widths either side of the spine. Smoothly relocate your knees into various areas of her back between her buttocks and shoulder, keeping your knees above her spinal column. Avoid the tendency to round your back during this technique, as you should keep your hara fully 'open' throughout.

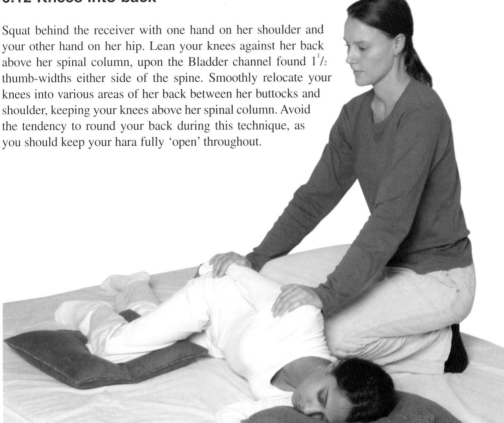

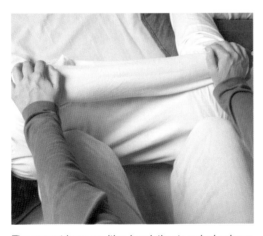

*The correct knee position in relation to spinal column.*

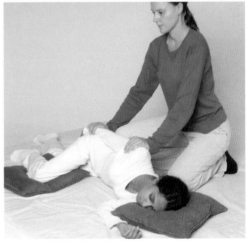

*VARIATION*
*If you find this technique difficult using both knees together, place one knee on the floor so that you are in squat kneeling and use one knee only on the receiver's back.*

## 6.13 Kneeling on bottom leg

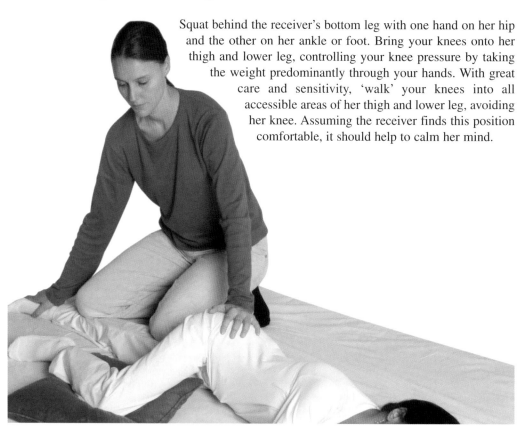

Squat behind the receiver's bottom leg with one hand on her hip and the other on her ankle or foot. Bring your knees onto her thigh and lower leg, controlling your knee pressure by taking the weight predominantly through your hands. With great care and sensitivity, 'walk' your knees into all accessible areas of her thigh and lower leg, avoiding her knee. Assuming the receiver finds this position comfortable, it should help to calm her mind.

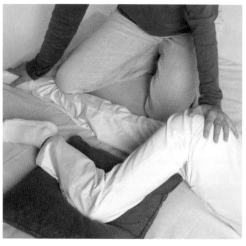

*VARIATION*
*If you find this technique difficult using both knees together, place one knee on the floor so that you are in squat kneeling and use one knee only on the receiver's leg.*

Note: If you find using even one knee too difficult, just palm down the receiver's leg.

## 6.14 Palming the hip, thigh and lower leg

Adopt the half kneeling stance behind the receiver, straddling her bottom leg. Placing one of your thumbs on top of the other, locate the centre of her buttock. Slowly lean enough pressure into this point for her to feel a definite sensation (leaning too hard will cause sharp pain). Adjust your position so that you have a support hand on her hip and then lean your other palm progressively down the outside of her thigh towards her knee. Finish the technique by adopting a wide kneeling stance and use both hands to palm along her lower leg.

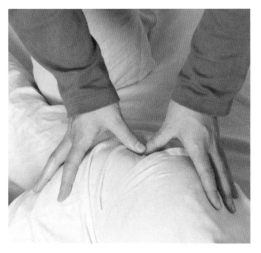

*1. Place one thumb on top of the other in the centre of the receiver's buttock and lean pressure into this point. Don't lean in too strongly.*

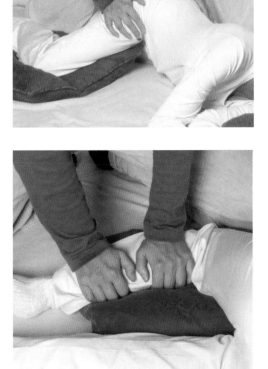

Now go back to the beginning of the side sequence and repeat all the techniques on the receiver's other side.

*2. Adopt wide kneeling stance and use both hands to palm along the lower leg.*

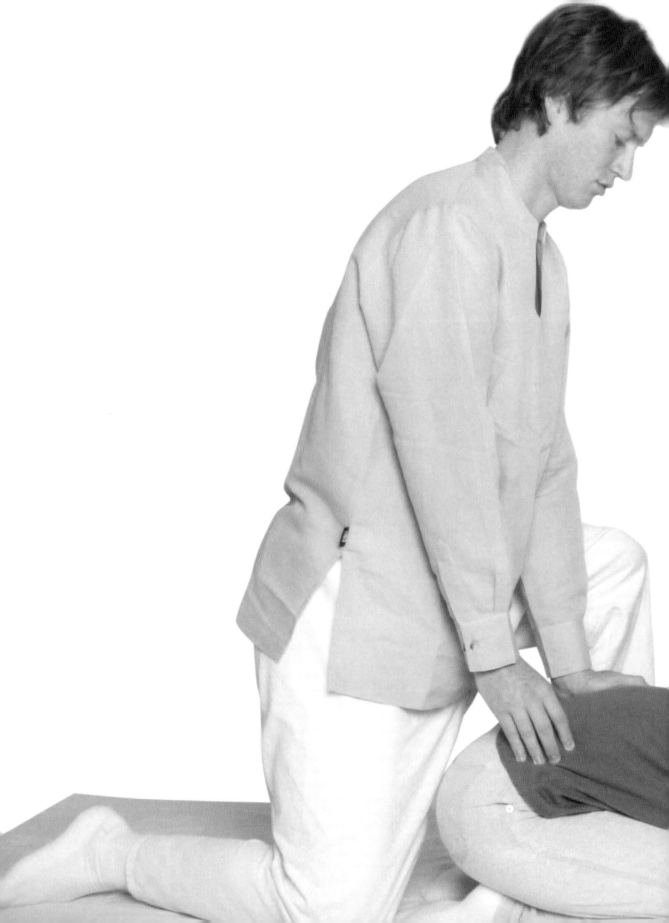

# CHAPTER 7

# Sitting Sequence

For these techniques, ask your receiver to kneel on the floor, or sit with crossed legs. Many people will find that the crossed leg position is more comfortable and easier to remain fully upright if they sit with buttocks raised up on a firm cushion or a foam block, 2–3 inches (5–7.5 cm) thick. In general, if your receiver is of similar height to you or smaller, you will find it easier to work on them if they kneel in seiza. If they are taller than you, it is usually easier to work on them if they sit with crossed legs. Many people will not be comfortable or able to sit in either position, in which case, many of the following techniques can be done with them seated on a stool.

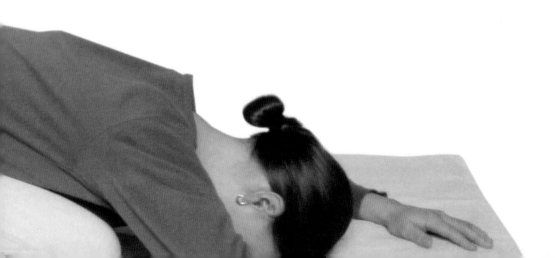

## 7.1 Palming down the spine

Kneel or squat kneel an arm's length behind the receiver. Place a support hand on her shoulder, close to the base of her neck (keep your fingers away from her throat). Leaning from your hara, use your other hand to palm down her back, either over her spine or to the side of the spine (the same side as the shoulder held by your support hand, as you will tend to twist her off balance if you palm the other side). Remember to keep your shoulders completely relaxed.

Repeat on the other side by placing your support hand on her other shoulder.

This is a good way to begin the sitting sequence because it enables you to feel easily whether or not the receiver is relaxed. It also encourages a better posture if she is slouching a little.

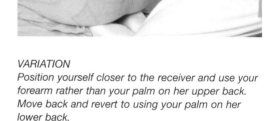

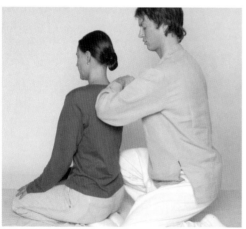

*VARIATION*
*Position yourself closer to the receiver and use your forearm rather than your palm on her upper back. Move back and revert to using your palm on her lower back.*

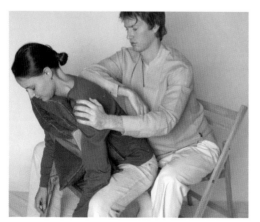

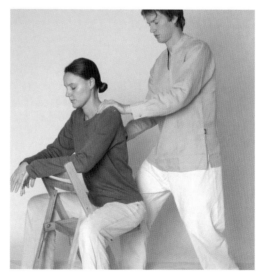

*Both variations of this technique can be carried out with the receiver seated on a chair or stool while the giver stands or also sits on a stool.*

## 7.2 Arm circling

In half kneeling beside and slightly behind the receiver, place your support hand over her shoulder. If you are able to find an indentation behind her shoulder, this is a good place to put your thumb. This indentation is a point called *Small Intestine 10*.

Now cradle her arm in yours and rotate her arm backwards in a way that resembles the arm movement of swimming backstroke. Make sure you pass her arm well in front of her torso, which reflects a natural movement for her shoulder joint. Repeat on the other arm.

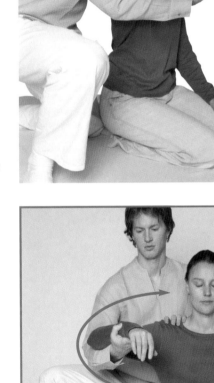

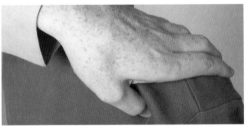

*Place your support hand on the receiver's shoulder with your thumb in the indentation behind the shoulder.*

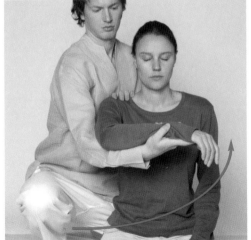

*Correct technique: the arm is passed well in front of the torso, reflecting the natural movement of the shoulder.*

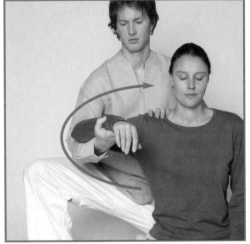

*Incorrect technique: the receiver's arm is not passed sufficiently across the front of her torso.*

Note: This technique can easily be applied with the receiver seated on a stool and the giver standing rather than kneeling. If the receiver has long arms, you may need to step forwards and then back again with your outside foot as you circle her arm.

## 7.3 Single arm overhead stretch

Progressing directly from Arm Circling, keep the same arm cradled in your arm and place your support hand on the receiver's other shoulder, close to the base of her neck. Bring her arm over her head, thus giving her inner arm and armpit a mild 'opening' stretch. Repeat on the other arm.

It is easy to cause damage to the shoulder if this technique is applied with too much zeal, so, as usual, never force; simply 'take up the slack'.

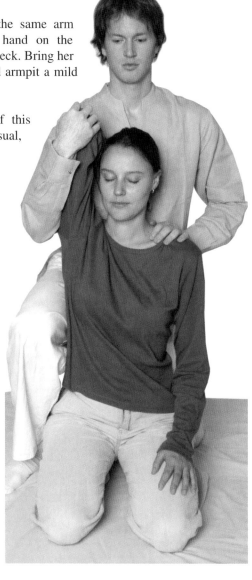

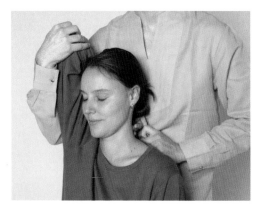

*VARIATION*
*A minor variation to this technique is to place one hand on the receiver's elbow and hold her hand with the other.*

## 7.4 Armpit/chest stretch

With the receiver clasping her hands behind her neck, stand behind her and hold her elbows. Ask her to allow her head to relax forwards naturally and encourage her to relax and release her whole upper body as you gently ease her elbows back. Keep your knees and thighs in contact with her back. Synchronize the opening of her chest with the rhythm of her exhalations, as this will make her feel she is in control of the stretch.

This technique helps to release stiffness in the muscles of the upper chest, expands the ribs and gently stretches the diaphragm. It therefore helps to improve breathing and posture. It also 'opens' the Heart channel, which runs along the inner surface of the arm from the armpit to the fifth finger. The Heart channel has a direct relationship with the mental focus, so if your receiver is a little sleepy this technique will perk her up. Conversely, if she is slightly agitated it may help to calm her.

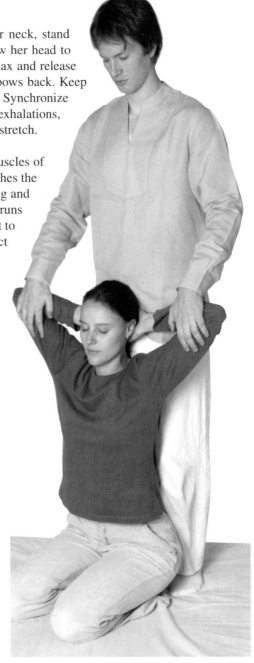

## 7.5 Forward neck stretch

In half kneeling beside the receiver, using your leg to support her back, rest her forehead in your palm. Place your other hand on the back of her neck. Ask her to 'give her head' to your palm, allowing her head to come forward progressively as she relaxes more. This will give a mild 'opening stretch' to the back of her neck. Now move her head and neck slightly from side to side, giving a mild stretch to the sides of her neck. Slowly bring her head back up, emphasizing that she should remain totally relaxed and not contribute any movement herself.

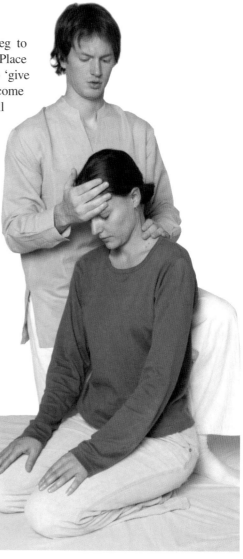

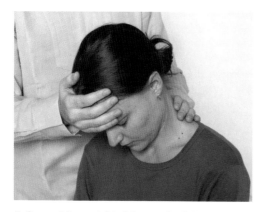

*1. Support the weight of the receiver's head as she relaxes it forward.*

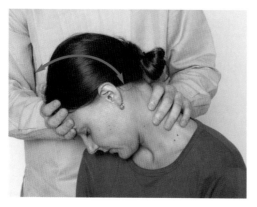

*2. Move her head slightly from side to side to give a stretch to the sides of her neck.*

Note: This technique should be done very slowly to avoid the receiver tensing up. If she has any neck problem, avoid the technique until you are more fully trained.

## 7.6 Child pose low back stretch

Have the receiver kneel with her head on the floor. If necessary she can raise her buttocks on a cushion. From standing or half kneeling, place one hand on one side of her lumbar area and the other hand on the opposite buttock. Apply a diagonal stretch. To develop your skill, try the movement using your forearms as well. Avoid leaning too high up her back because that will compress her neck and squash her face into the floor.

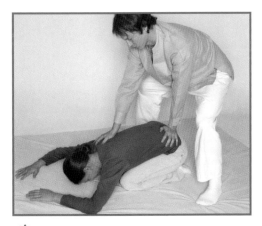

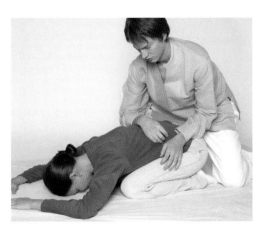

*As an alternative to using your hands, try using your forearms.*

*Incorrect technique: if your hands are placed too high up the receiver's back, you will compress her neck and squash her face into the floor.*

## 7.7 Back dispersal

This technique can be done with the receiver kneeling with her head on the floor or sitting or kneeling upright. Vigorously disperse tension and stiffness from the hip and buttock area with the heel of your hand or your fingertips. Alternatively, use hacking, cupping, or closed palm cushioning (see below), in which case you should avoid the kidney area. Repeat on the shoulder blade area.

This type of 'back dispersal' technique is more common within other forms of oriental bodywork. However, it is a good instant remedy for the receiver if she feels stiff around the hips, buttocks or shoulder blades after a prolonged period of sitting.

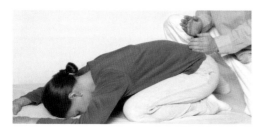

Hacking (chopping with the heel of your hand) on the buttock area.

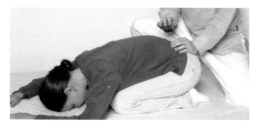

Cupping (slapping with hollowed palms) on the buttock area.

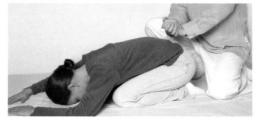

Closed palm cushioning (palms held loosely together).

## 7.8 Hara/sacrum support

In this technique the receiver kneels or sits upright. Kneel beside her, facing her side. Hold her hara and sacrum simultaneously, tuning into her breathing rhythm.

This is a good way to finish the sitting sequence and indeed this beginner's sequence as a whole. Holding the hara and sacrum is very energizing for the receiver because you are helping her to become more aware of this area through making contact with her centre – the core of her body and the source of her vitality.

When you remove your hands very slowly to finish, the receiver will be so focused on her belly that she will experience a sensation akin to your hands being still in place. This indicates that her mind is now more attuned with the sensations of her body.

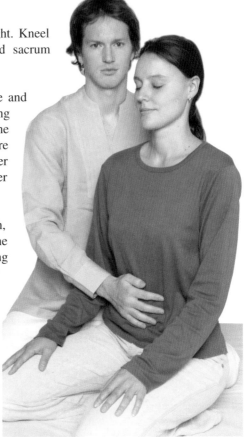

# CHAPTER 8

# Oriental Medicine Theory For Basic Shiatsu

The most basic level of shiatsu can be applied without reference to any detailed Oriental medicine theory. All that is required is an experiential understanding of the information described in this book so far; along with some degree of skill acquired through repetitive practice. A course of shiatsu study of around 10–12 days or so (including some basic musculo-skeletal anatomy), spread over a few months, would bring you up to that level. However, your understanding and appreciation of what shiatsu is capable of will be enhanced enormously if you learn some simple rudiments of Oriental medicine theory, as presented in this chapter.

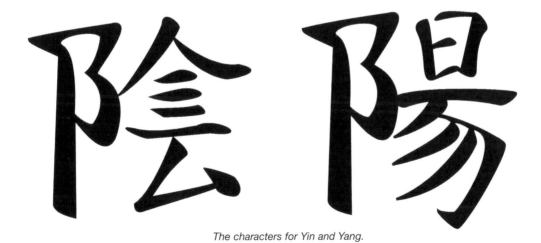

*The characters for Yin and Yang.*

# Yin-Yang Theory

Shiatsu is all about encouraging harmony and balance within the receiver's body and mind, primarily through optimising their Ki. The concept of harmony and balance in traditional oriental philosophy is expressed through the idea of *Yin / Yang*. Yin / Yang is basically the polarity that exists within and between everything that exists. This means that all things are perceived in relation to their opposite. For example, hot is only hot because we have the concept of cold, and vice-versa, neither of which can exist without the other. As such, everything in nature has both Yin and Yang qualities – nothing is totally one or the other. This means that things can only be described as *more* Yin or *less* Yin, or *more* Yang or *less* Yang, than something else. Warm water for example, is more Yang than ice but more Yin compared to steam. You can never say that something is completely Yang or Yin because nothing is really fixed or unchangeable in nature; for example, big can always be bigger and small can always be smaller.

The starting point for differentiating more Yin qualities from more Yang qualities began several thousand years ago by attributing heat to Yang and cold to Yin. Thereafter, the qualities associated with Yin are described as analogous to those phenomena that predominate on the shady, cooler side of a hill. By contrast, Yang qualities are associated with those phenomena observed on the sunny, warmer side of a hill. Leading on from that, the ancient Daoist philosophers attributed other things with relative Yin or Yang qualities by observing natural phenomena occurring on either side of the hill. Many of their comparisons of Yin / Yang are listed below:

| In the Yin category | In the Yang category |
| --- | --- |
| Darkness | Light |
| Cold | Heat |
| Rest | Movement |
| Wet | Dry |

Yin and Yang are therefore inextricably related; they are opposing but also complementary. The two make up the full picture; without the one the other is incomplete. The Yin / Yang symbol actually embodies the complete philosophy of Yin / Yang.

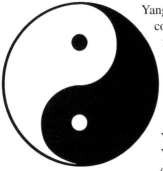

Yang is the white part of the symbol and Yin is the black part. The two components coil around each other, they penetrate each other, they fade into one another. They are opposites yet they complement one another. The white part of the symbol contains a black spot and the black part a white spot, signifying that nothing is ever entirely Yin or Yang but each contains something of the other, which may grow so that eventually each can become its opposite.

Yin and Yang phenomena can themselves be further divided into Yin and Yang. For example day is Yang compared to night, but a day may be divided into morning and afternoon. Morning, when the sun is rising, is more Yang than the afternoon, when the sun is setting, so morning is more Yang and afternoon is more Yin.

*Yin and Yang symbol.*

Morning turns into afternoon, which can therefore be expressed as Yang turning into Yin. Day becomes night, summer turns to winter, our bodies move then rest, we are warm then cool, and we wake then sleep. The movement from Yin to Yang is cyclical.

In general, you will see that phenomena which is non-material, more refined, less tangible, and energetic rather than solid is Yang in relation to what is solid, material, grosser and tangible, which is Yin. With that in mind we can add anything to the 'more Yin, more Yang list', such as the examples given opposite:

If we contemplate the idea of Yin / Yang, we can see that there are five main ways in which they are related to each another: they oppose one another; they complement one another; they can consume one another; they can transform into one another. In addition they are infinitely divisible.

| Yin | Yang |
| --- | --- |
| Dark | Light |
| Cold | Heat |
| Rest | Movement |
| Wet | Dry |
| Moon | Sun |
| Earth | Heaven |
| West | East |
| North | South |
| Matter/substance | Energy/thought |
| Solid/liquid | Vapour/gas |
| Solidifying | Dissolving |
| Condensation | Evaporation |
| Contraction | Expansion |
| Descending | Rising |
| Below | Above |
| Form | Activity |
| Water | Fire |
| Yielding | Resistant |
| Passive | Aggressive |
| Introverted | Outgoing |
| Quiet | Loud |
| Slow | Fast |
| Chronic | Acute |
| Curves | Straight lines |
| Feminine | Masculine |

*1. Yin and Yang are opposites.*

Therefore they struggle against one another and keep one another in check. Cold cools down heat: cooling drinks refresh on a hot day. Heat warms up cold: a fire heats you up on a cold day.

This is the basis of treatment in Oriental medicine: if you have a hot condition, treatment should be cooling and vice-versa. Treatment opposes one force with a contrary one.

The struggle between Yin and Yang results in a state of dynamic balance. In the body as in other spheres the balance is constantly changing. Take body temperature: it is basically stable, but within a certain narrow range it fluctuates. If it fluctuates beyond that particular range, the physiological balance of the body is lost and dis-ease arises.

*2. Yin and Yang are interdependent.*

Yin and Yang are opposed to each other and interdependent at the same time. For example, daytime is Yang, but daytime depends on the existence of night, which is Yin. Hence, we experience the continuous cycle of alternating day and night. Even if the earth stopped spinning, half the planet would be in perpetual day balanced by the other half in perpetual night. Also consider going up or coming down. You can only go up (Yang) if there is a down (Yin) and vice-versa. In the vast emptiness of deep space, you would have no perception of which way you were going, as there would be no obvious point of reference. You need to be moving in relation to something to experience movement.

*3. Yin and Yang tend to consume one another.*

This means that where Yin predominates it will overwhelm and use up Yang and vice-versa. For the body to work normally and keep itself warm (Yang), it has to burn up part of its substance (Yin). On the other hand producing nutrient substances for the body (Yin) consumes a bit of energy (Yang). If either the Yin or Yang aspects of the body go beyond the normal range, the result is either an excess or a deficiency of one or the other; resulting in disease.

*4. Yin and Yang can transform into one another.*

Yin will transform into Yang and vice-versa when either Yin or Yang reach an extreme. For example, very cold water is more Yin in temperature than moderately cold water, but freezing water is so cold (Yin) that it changes quality and turns to ice. Ice expands and floats on water because it becomes less dense than water, thereby taking on Yang attributes (expansion and decrease in density are both Yang qualities). Conversely, extreme heat (hot = Yang) causes water (cool = Yin) to expand into steam (expanded = Yang) that rises (upward = Yang). At altitude the steam cools and condenses back to water (cool and condenses = Yin), which then falls to earth as rain (downward = Yin). To quote from an ancient Daoist text called the *Su Wen*; "*Extreme cold will bring about heat, and extreme heat will induce cold...*"

*5. Yin and Yang can be further divided into Yin and Yang.*

I gave the example earlier about day dividing further into morning and afternoon. Likewise one can divide the year into summer (Yang) and winter (Yin), or further into summer (Yang within Yang), autumn (Yin within (*coming out of*) Yang), winter (Yin within Yin) and spring (Yang within (*coming out of*) Yin).

**The Correspondences of Yin-Yang Within the Body**

What is more relevant to the professional shiatsu therapist, is how Yin / Yang can be differentiated in the human body, as outlined in the following table:

| Yin | | Yang |
|---|---|---|
| | *Anatomy:* | |
| Lower part (body) | | Upper part (head) |
| Interior (internal organs) | | Exterior (skin, muscles) |
| Medial (Yin channels) | | Lateral (Yang channels) |
| Front (Yin channels) | | Back (Yang channels) |
| | *Physiology:* | |
| Substance | | Activity |
| Store vital substances | | Digest and excrete |
| Blood and body fluids | | Ki |
| Down-bearing | | Upward-moving |
| Inward movement | | Outward movement |
| Yin moves energy ... | | Yang moves energy ... |
| (... and substances down to anus and urethra) | | (... and substances out to skin and limbs) |

*Pathology:*

| | |
|---|---|
| Cold (feelings of cold, aversion to cold, chills) | Hot (feelings of heat, aversion to heat, fever) |
| Quiet (sleepiness, aversion to movement/talking) | Restless (insomnia, tremors, fidgeting) |
| Wet (watery eyes, runny nose, loose stools, discharges) | Dry (eyes, nose, mouth, stools) |
| Soft (lumps and swellings) | Hard (lumps and swellings) |
| Inhibition (hypoactivity) | Excitement (hyperactivity) |
| Slowness (movement, speech) | Rapidity (movement, speech) |
| Chronic disease | Acute disease |
| Gradual onset | Rapid onset |
| Lingering disease | Rapid changes |
| Likes to be covered | Throws off blankets |
| Pale face | Red face |
| Shallow breathing | Coarse breathing |

## Yin-Yang as a Guide to Diagnosis and Treatment

The root cause of any disease is an imbalance between Yin and Yang. The basic principle of Oriental medicine and of shiatsu is to adjust Yin and Yang in order to restore harmony of body and mind. If we can understand the nature of the imbalance correctly we can take the appropriate steps to correct it. Balancing Kyo and Jitsu directly within the Ki channels (see pages 13–17) is the shiatsu practitioner's primary method of restoring the Yin / Yang balance of the recipient. Kyo has several Yin qualities such as deeper; more hidden; underlying and more slow to respond to treatment. Jitsu has more Yang qualities such as appearing more obvious and quicker to respond to treatment. Kyo and Jitsu always exist together at some level within the person.

Another method that can be used by the shiatsu practitioner to influence the Yin / Yang ratios in the body is through the use of specific tsubos that have documented effects upon the body's Yin / Yang ratio. Ideally, this approach is better applied in tandem with herbal medicine and dietary advice. Through various methods of diagnosis, the practitioner will assess the person as having insufficient Yang (Empty Yang), too much Yang (Excess Yang), insufficient Yin (Empty Yin), or too much Yin (Excess Yin).

Excess Yang causes the body to generate heat and become overactive. However, heat and dryness can be generated because of a lack of cool, moist Yin quality in the body, allowing the hotter Yang to predominate. This is Empty Yin. Empty Yang results in coldness and lethargy. Excess Yin is comparatively rare as it can only occur from exposure to extreme cold, so it is not shown on the diagram overleaf, which illustrates these comparisons.

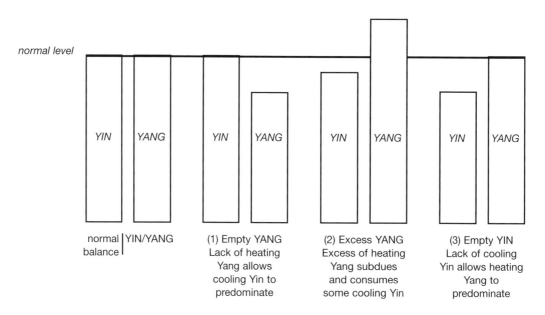

*normal level*

| normal balance | YIN/YANG | (1) Empty YANG Lack of heating Yang allows cooling Yin to predominate | (2) Excess YANG Excess of heating Yang subdues and consumes some cooling Yin | (3) Empty YIN Lack of cooling Yin allows heating Yang to predominate |

*Yin/Yang combinations.*

## Five Element Theory

From Yin-Yang theory it is clear that the ancient Chinese view of the universe focuses on the harmonious balance achieved through the perpetual movement and ever changing nature of phenomena. It is not a static view, but one of dynamic movement. Yin and Yang maintain a dynamic balance between one another. *Five-Element theory* or *Five-Phase theory*, as it is also called, is another part of this view of change and movement. According to this idea, all phenomena are products of the movement of five qualities: water, wood, fire, earth, and metal. These elements or phases are not the fundamental components of matter, but rather they are descriptions of certain qualities that pertain to particular phases of change.

### The most commonly used correspondences

Each Element stands for many related qualities and correspondences. All phenomena can be classified according to the Five Elements: planets, animals, directions, seasons, sounds, odours, and emotions (see table opposite).

### Water
Water is associated with the very Yin qualities of winter, night and with rest. It gives us the will to live (called *Zhi*), the most basic human drive, and the urge to procreate. It relates to the Kidney that houses the will and stores the Essence, the basis of our constitutional strength. The Bladder also belongs to the Water Element. Fear is the emotion associated with Water. A bluish or black tinge to the face, especially below the eyes, a groaning quality to the voice and a putrid odour may manifest with a Water imbalance. A person with a predominance of Water may be self-possessed and able, but may become timid or fearful if the Water Element is unbalanced.

| | WATER | WOOD | FIRE | EARTH | METAL |
|---|---|---|---|---|---|
| Direction | North | East | South | Centre | West |
| Season | Winter | Spring | Summer | Late summer | Autumn |
| Climate | Cold | Wind | Heat | Dampness | Dryness |
| Process | Storage | Birth | Growth | Transforming | Gathering in |
| Activity | Rest | Initiating | Peak | Balance | Decline |
| Time | Night | Morning | Noon | Late afternoon | Evening |
| Colour | Blue/black | Green | Red | Yellow | White |
| Taste | Salty | Sour | Bitter | Sweet | Pungent |
| Smell | Rotten | Rancid | Scorched | Fragrant | Musty |
| Zang | Kidney | Liver | Heart/ Heart Protector | Spleen | Lung |
| Fu | Bladder | Gallbladder | Small Intestine/ Triple Heater | Stomach | Large Intestine |
| Sense organ | Ears | Eyes | Tongue | Mouth | Nose |
| Tissue | Bones | Tendons/ ligaments | Blood vessels | Flesh | Skin/ body hair |
| Body Fluid | Urine | Tears | Sweat | Saliva | Mucus |
| Emotion | Fear | Anger | Joy | Worry/ pensiveness | Grief |
| Sound | Groaning | Shouting | Laughter | Singing | Weeping |
| Mind | Endurance/ will | Planning/ controlling | Love/ sensitivity | Concentration/ analysing | Taking in/ letting go |
| Spiritual | Willpower/ Zhi | Ethereal soul/ Hun | Consciousness/ Shen | Intellect/ Yi | Corporeal soul/ Po |
| Energetic directions in Cosmological Cycle | Downwards | Expansion | Upward | Centre, stability | Contraction |
| Energetic directions in the Creation and Controlling Cycles | Floating or suspended | Rising | Expanding, radiating in all directions | Descending | Meeting |

## Wood

Wood is associated with the more Yang qualities of spring, morning and with initiating action. It gives the ability to plan, control, assert and to be angry. It relates to the Liver and Gallbladder. The Liver houses the Ethereal Soul, which the Chinese call the *Hun*. The Hun leaves the body at death and is considered the source of hope and vision. A loud, shouting or clipped voice, a greenish tinged complexion and a rancid odour may manifest with a Wood imbalance. People with a predominance of Wood are usually assertive, authoritative and well organized, but may be irritable.

### Fire

Fire is associated with the very Yang qualities of summer, noon and with peak activity. It gives us the capacity for warmth and love. It relates to the Heart and Small Intestine and the Heart Protector and Triple Heater. The Heart houses the mind, the seat of consciousness, the origin of all thought and emotion. The consciousness in Chinese medicine is called the *Shen*. A reddish complexion, a laughing or tremulous voice and a scorched odour may manifest with a Fire imbalance. A person with a predominance of Fire is often warm and sensitive but may also be excitable and emotionally changeable.

### Earth

Earth is associated with late summer, late afternoon and decreasing activity, which are qualities of Yin arising as Yang subsides. It gives us the capacity for intellectual thought and concentration (called *Yi*), and for pensiveness and sympathy. It relates to the Spleen and Stomach and so to nourishment: i.e. the taking in and digestion of food and information, both physically and intellectually. A yellowish tinge to the complexion, a singing quality to the voice and a slightly sickly-sweet odour may manifest with an Earth imbalance. People with a predominance of Earth are often good and sympathetic listeners, but may have a tendency to worry.

### Metal

Metal is associated with the relatively Yin qualities of autumn, evening and with the balance between activity and rest. It gives us the capacity to take in new experience and to eliminate and let go of the old. It relates to the Lung and Large Intestine. The Lung houses the Corporeal Soul (called *P'o*), which gives us animal vitality and the ability to live in the present. Grief and sadness relate to Metal. The skin is an extension of the Lung, so the Metal element is associated with the idea of boundary, of the border between others and us. A whitish tinge to the face, a weeping quality to the voice and a rather musty odour of decay may manifest with a Metal imbalance. People with a predominance of Metal can be very 'present' and optimistic, or may easily feel 'invaded' or melancholic.

On the whole, people do not fall neatly into a single category but tend to combine qualities from a number of different Elements. They may, however, exhibit a predominance of a particular element at a given time, or over their lifetime.

The Five Elements interact in three natural ways that are relevant to Oriental medicine. These are known as the *Cosmological cycle*, the *Creation cycle* and the *Controlling cycle*. To this we can add the *Rebelling* or *Insulting cycle*, which depicts what happens when their harmony is compromised. These cycles are represented in the following diagrams.

**The Cosmological Cycle**

The Cosmological cycle is the first known reference to the Five Elements. And the Elements were listed as follows: water, fire, wood, metal and earth. It is represented as follows:

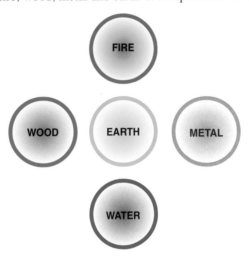

Water is the first mentioned Element and is placed at the bottom: it is the basis of the sequence, the foundation of all the other elements. This concept is central to Oriental medical thinking: Water and specifically the Kidneys are the root of Yin and Yang, the foundation of all the other organs, the starting point of good health. Fire is placed opposite Water, at the top of the cycle. This reflects the fundamental opposition of Yin and Yang and the idea that Fire and Water oppose yet balance one another. There is direct communication between Water below and Fire above, as they are at the two extremities of a common axis. This idea translates in medical terms into the notion that Yin Water must flow upward to nourish the Heart, while the Fire of the Heart must flow downward to warm the Kidneys; also Essence must be strong (Kidneys and Water) for the Mind (Heart and Fire) to flourish.

In the centre, is Earth. The Stomach and Spleen play the principle role in nourishing all the organs, because they digest food and provide Ki for the body. The Heart especially relies on them to provide Ki for the production and pumping of Blood. So the Stomach and Spleen are considered to be the main source of Ki and Blood produced after birth from food and air, called the *Post-Heaven Ki*. Therefore whenever there is deficiency of Ki and Blood in the body, it may be useful to tonify and strengthen the Earth Element in order to provide Ki and Blood for other organs.

Finally this arrangement of Fire, Earth and Water reflects the idea of heaven above, earth below and human beings in the Centre, which is central to the oriental view of the universe.

## The Creation Cycle

The diagram below represents the Creation cycle, also known as the *Generating cycle* or the *Shen cycle*. In the Creation cycle each Element creates or generates the one that succeeds it in the cycle and is in turn created by the one that precedes it. This is known as *Mother-Child relationship* between Elements. Each Element is the mother of its succeeding Element and the child of its preceding one.

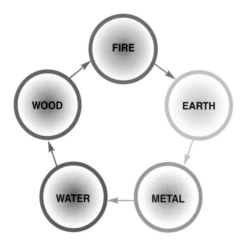

- Water nourishes Wood so it is the Mother of Wood; it is also the Child of Metal.
- Wood burns so it is said to be the Mother of Fire; it is also the Child of Water.
- Fire creates ashes so it is said to be the Mother of Earth; it is also the Child of Wood.
- Earth contains metal ores so it is said to be the Mother of Metal; it is also the Child of Fire.
- Metal melts (becomes liquid) so it is said to be the Mother of Water; it is also the Child of Earth.

## The Controlling Cycle

The diagram below depicts the Controlling cycle, also known as the *Restraining cycle* or the *Ko cycle*. In this cycle each element controls or restrains the next but one in the cycle and is controlled by the one-before-the-one-before it.

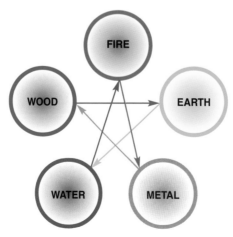

- Wood penetrates Earth so Wood is said to control Earth *(plant roots binding soil together)*.

- Earth channels Water so Earth is said to control Water *(rivers and lakes are contained by their surrounding earth banks)*.

- Water extinguishes Fire so Water is said to control Fire.

- Fire melts Metal so Fire is said to control Metal.

- Metal cuts Wood so Metal is said to control Wood.

If any element is excessive or deficient, this will in turn affect other Elements along one or the other, or indeed both, cycles.

If the effect of imbalance is felt along the creation cycle, then either the Mother or the Child Element is affected; this can be either the Mother affecting the Child or conversely the Child affecting the Mother. The Mother can affect the Child by not nourishing it enough. The Child can affect the Mother by drawing too much from her and weakening her.

If the effect of imbalance is felt along the controlling cycle it can result in "overacting" or over-controlling of one Element by another. This follows the normal cycle, but is simply an excess of controlling. For example, Fire normally controls Metal, but if Fire is excessive it can act too powerfully upon Metal and damage it. This is overacting, also sometimes called *invading*.

**The Rebelling Cycle**

The counteracting or rebelling (also called *insulting*) cycle is the other effect that can occur along the controlling cycle. This occurs when the controlling cycle goes into reverse at some point, i.e. the controlling cycle flows backwards. For example Fire controls Metal but if Fire is weak and Metal is strong then Metal can attack Fire instead of being controlled by it.

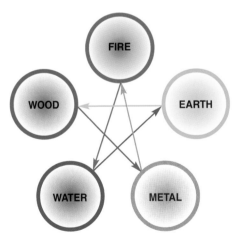

So if an element is in excess, it will tend to overact on the element it usually controls, and it will also tend to rebel against the element that usually controls it.

The following diagram illustrates the internal organs and seasons in relation to the Five Elements in the Creation, Controlling and Rebelling cycles.

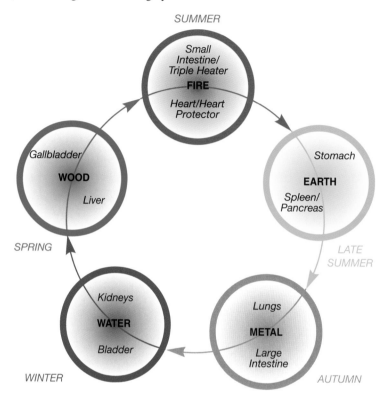

## Practical Application

In terms of the practical application of Five Element theory, many of the correspondences are useful clinically. Taking Wood and the Liver as an example: people with Liver imbalances (in the Oriental medicine sense of Ki imbalance, rather than the Western physiological sense) will often have a greenish tinge to their complexion, their voice may also be quite loud, they may be irritable and worse for windy weather.

The eyes relate to Liver, but it is not the only organ that can affect the eyes. The Heart channel has an internal branch which goes to the eyes, the Gallbladder and Triple Heater channels begin and end respectively near the eyes, and indeed problems unrelated to internal organ pathology may affect the eyes. In other words, although Five Element theory says that the eyes relate to Liver, clinically the facts are more complicated. The model has its limitations. It is therefore unwise to rely on the Five Element model of correspondences alone for diagnosis.

The cosmological, creation and controlling cycles provide a model of a dynamic balance between the elements. If the balance is upset, disease ensues. If the cosmological cycle is affected and if the Kidneys (Water) are weak, this will directly affect both the Spleen (Earth) and the Heart (Fire), causing weakness in one or both. In the case of the creation cycle, if the Kidneys are weak, this will impact on the Liver (Wood), causing deficiency. In the case of the controlling cycle if the Ki of the Liver stagnates it may overact on the Spleen, disrupting digestion. This is called Liver invading the Spleen and it is a commonly seen pattern. However, Lungs overacting on Liver is not a common pattern. In other words the model may be a useful tool to interpret some clinical facts, but should not be applied too rigidly.

For the shiatsu therapist, the Five Element model is useful insofar as it can help them understand the reason behind their diagnosis. In some situations, it can also influence their treatment strategy.

## The Internal Organs (Zangfu)

Most Channels are named after an organ. However, the Oriental medical view of each organ is wider in connotation than in Western medicine. Try not to equate these functions with the Western concept of organ function. That will only lead to total confusion. The term for *Organ* as defined by Traditional Oriental Medicine is *Zangfu*.

The twelve Zangfu Organs are classified in pairs. Each pair contains one Yin (or *Zang*) and one Yang (or *Fu*) Organ. Thus we have six pairs of Zangfu.

| Yin (Zang) Organ | Yang (Fu) Organ |
| --- | --- |
| Kidneys | Bladder |
| Liver | Gallbladder |
| Heart | Small Intestines |
| Heart Protector | Triple Heater |
| Spleen | Stomach |
| Lungs | Large Intestines |

When referring to organs in Oriental medicine we will use a capital letter to differentiate them from the Western meanings, e.g. Kidneys, Heart, etc. The same applies to any other concepts, which may take on a slightly different meaning from that which you are used to in everyday language, e.g. Blood, Body Fluids.

Oriental medicine describes each Organ and its functions in relation to: a) Ki, Blood, and Body Fluids; b) a specific body tissue; c) a sense organ; d) an emotion; e) a climate. The following few pages describe these relationships.

## The Internal Organs in Relation to Ki

*The Kidneys Store Ki as 'Essence', and Control the Reception of Ki*

The Kidneys store Ki as 'Essence', which is a 'denser', more Yin state of Ki, responsible for growth and reproduction. Most of this Essence is inherited from our parents, but can be supplemented by Ki extracted from food by the Spleen.

The Kidneys anchor the Ki extracted from air by the Lungs. If the Kidneys fail to do this, Ki will become trapped in the chest and asthma may develop.

The Liver ensures that Ki flows smoothly through the Channels and to the organs. If it fails to do this, Ki stagnates, obstructing the body functions and causing the mind to become tense and frustrated. On the other hand, tension and frustration can block Ki flow and upset the Liver.

*The Spleen Extracts Ki from Food*

When food is ingested, the Spleen extracts Ki from it. This process intimately involves the Stomach; because the Stomach is said to 'rot and ripen' ingested food, meaning that it prepares it for Ki extraction by the Spleen. The Spleen sends some of this Food-Ki to the Lungs to combine with Ki extracted from air, which is then circulated through the Channels, and under the skin as Defensive Ki. The Spleen also sends some Food-Ki to the Heart to enrich the Blood and give it impetus.

*The Lungs Govern Ki and Respiration*

When air is inhaled, the Lungs extract fresh 'pure' Ki from it. On exhalation, stale Ki is expelled, along with waste gases. This maintains the continual renewal and freshness of bodily Ki.

Ki extracted from food by the Spleen combines with the Ki from air to be circulated through the Channels. It is also circulated under the skin as Defensive Ki (protecting us from weather extremes and pathogenic organisms, and also warming the skin and muscles).

The Large Intestine also has a role in the formation of Defensive Ki. The Lungs also send Ki downwards for the Kidneys to 'grasp', and provide Ki for the functioning of the Bladder and Large Intestine.

## The Internal Organs in Relation to Blood

*The Liver Stores Blood*

The Liver regulates the amount of Blood in circulation according to the levels of physical activity. During rest, a large proportion of Blood flows to the Liver to be stored. During physical activity, the Blood returns to general circulation, ensuring adequate energy, and nourishing of the joints, skin, nails and other body parts.

*The Heart Governs Blood*

This means that if the Heart is strong, it can pump Blood efficiently and in abundance throughout the body. Therefore, it plays the major role in circulation. The Heart Protector assists the Heart in this function. The Lungs also assist the Heart in this function by providing Ki for the propulsion of blood and for the maintenance of blood vessels.

*The Spleen is the Source of Blood, and Holds Blood*

Because the Spleen is the main organ of digestion, it helps transform ingested food and drink into Blood. It 'controls' Blood by keeping it in the blood vessels (by transforming nutrients into healthy blood vessels). Failure of this function can result in haemorrhage or excessive menstrual bleeding.

## The Internal Organs in Relation to Body Fluids

*The Kidneys Govern Water*

The Kidneys may be thought of as a 'gate', which opens and closes to control the flow of fluid secretion. When the warming, more energizing function of the Kidneys (Kidney-Yang) is deficient, the gate is too open, leading to copious, clear urination. When the cooling, more nourishing function of the Kidneys (Kidney-Yin) is deficient, the gate is too closed, leading to scanty, dark urination.

The Bladder physically performs the storage and excretion of urine, although it is the Kidneys, which provide the energy (Ki) to transform bodily fluids into urine.

### The Heart Controls Sweat

Body Fluids enter the blood vessels to thin down the Blood when it gets too thick. Conversely, Body Fluids leave the Blood if the Blood gets too thin. Thus there is a constant interchange between Blood and Body Fluids. The heart controls this function. Continuous excessive sweating will therefore lead to a loss of Body Fluids and consequent deficiency of Blood. Weakness in the Heart-Ki may result in spontaneous sweating.

### The Spleen Separates and Transports Fluids

The Spleen separates the usable part of ingested fluids from the unusable part. The usable or 'clean' part goes upwards to the Lungs for distribution to the skin. The unusable or 'dirty' part goes downwards to the Small Intestine for further refinement. If this function of the Spleen is impaired, the fluids may accumulate to create Dampness, too much Phlegm, or cause water retention (oedema).

The Stomach assists the Spleen in the extraction of fluids from food to make Body Fluids.

### The Lungs Disperse Body Fluids and Regulate Water Passages

The Lungs influence the excretion of sweat and urine. Firstly, they spread Body Fluids all over the body to the skin, moistening it, and regulating the opening and closing of the pores. As such, the Lungs influence sweating. Water retention (oedema) in the face may result if this function is impaired. The Lungs also help the Bladder's function of excreting urine.

## The Internal Organs in Relation to the Tissues

### The Kidneys Control the Bones and Manifest in the Hair

The strength and growth of bones depends on the strength of the Essence, which enables growth. Because the Kidneys store this Essence (which equates with the genetic structure of the body) they therefore control the bones and teeth. The bone marrow, in Oriental medicine, includes the brain, spinal cord, and nerves. Thus, the Kidneys control these also.

The hair on the head also depends upon the Essence and therefore the Kidneys for normal growth. Weak Essence reflects in thin, brittle and greying hair.

### The Liver Controls the Sinews and Manifests in the Nails

Because the Liver regulates the amount of Blood in circulation, it controls the nourishment of the tendons and ligaments, ensuring smooth movement of joints and ease of muscular action. Failure of the Liver function results in stiffness, or even tremors. The Gallbladder also relates to the sinews. Whereas the Liver nourishes the sinews and Blood, The Gallbladder provides them with sufficient Ki to ensure their proper movement. The Liver's regulation of Blood also determines the amount of nourishment reaching the nails. A lack of Blood in circulation therefore results in cracked, dry and indented nails.

*The Heart Controls the Blood Vessels and Manifests in the Complexion*

As part of its function of governing the Blood, the Heart also controls the strength of contraction of the blood vessels. A healthy Heart will mean strong blood vessels, healthy circulation, and consequently a lustrous, rosy complexion.

*The Spleen Controls the Muscles and Manifests in the Lips*

The Spleen extracts nourishment from the food and transports it to the body parts, including the muscles, ensuring their strength and development.

Food passing the lips is the first stage of digestion. For this reason, the lips are closely connected to the Spleen. Therefore dry, cracked or pale lips show that Spleen-Ki is weak.

*The Lungs Control the Skin and Body Hair*

Because the Lungs disperse Ki to the skin and ensure that the body surface receives adequate nourishment and moisture, the Lungs are said to control the skin and body hair. If the Body Fluids are properly dispersed by the Lungs, the skin will be lustrous and the hair shiny. If not, the skin will become dry and body hair brittle and withered.

## The Internal Organs and the Sense Organs

*The Kidneys Control the Ears and Hearing*

The Essence, which is stored in the Kidneys to enable growth and reproduction, is also required to enable the ears to function. Therefore the ears and hearing relate most closely to the Kidneys.

*The Liver Controls the Eyes and Sight*

The Liver nourishes and maintains the eyes because it regulates the amount of Blood in circulation, and because a deep pathway of the Liver channel enters the eyes. If this Liver function is impaired, there may be dry, gritty eyes, poor vision and the presence of spots or 'floaters'. However, many other organs also influence the eyes.

*The Heart Controls the Tongue and Taste*

Although the tongue shows the condition of all the Organs, it has particular bearing on that of the Heart, because a deep pathway of the Heart channel enters the tongue. The Heart therefore controls the sense of taste and affects speech.

*The Spleen Controls the Mouth and Taste*

The Spleen influences the sense of taste as well as a feeling of appetite. It relates to the mouth because chewing is the first stage in the transformation of food. Food transformation is a function of the Spleen, assisted by the Stomach.

*The Lungs Control the Nose and Smell*

The Lungs are intimately connected with the breath. The nose is the gateway of the breath. Therefore the Lungs control the nose and the sense of smell. However, the Spleen also influences smell. The nose becomes blocked when the Ki of the Lungs is weak.

**The Internal Organs and Mental Faculties**

*The Kidneys House Willpower*

The willpower, which is under the influence of the Kidneys, provides the instinct for survival, determination and the drive to procreate. The emotion related to the Kidneys is fear.

The Gallbladder also has an influence on willpower and drive insofar as it gives the courage and initiative to turn the Kidneys' drive into decisive action.

*The Liver Houses the Ethereal Soul*

The ethereal soul is the part of one's being considered to survive after death to return to the world of immaterial existence. During life it provides us with our capacity for vision and planning. The emotion related to the Liver is anger.

The Liver is paired with the Gallbladder, which controls judgement and the capacity to make decisions. Decision-making is also influenced by the Small Intestine. Whereas the Gallbladder gives us the courage and initiative to make decisions, it is the Small Intestine which provides the clarity of mind to make decisions.

*The Heart Houses the Mind*

The Heart influences the Mind, in that it governs mental activity, emotions, consciousness, memory, thinking and sleep. This is because the Heart controls the Blood. When Blood is abundant and freely circulating to all the Organs and the brain, the mental faculties are clear. This function of influencing the Mind is shared with the Heart Protector. However, although the Heart and Heart Protector govern the broad spectrum of Mind functions, the other Organs influence aspects of these functions, as described below. The emotion related to the Heart is joy.

*The Spleen Houses Thought*

The Spleen influences the process of thinking, analyzing, concentrating and studying, ensuring strong powers of reasoning and memory. A weakness in the Spleen-Ki will result in unclear thought processes and over thinking. The emotion related to the Spleen is pensiveness and worry.

*The Lungs House the Corporeal Soul*

The corporeal soul is that which enables us to feel sensations. Consequently it is the most physical and material aspect of our 'soul'. Since it deals with sensations felt in the present, it enables us to experience 'reality' which is the sum total of experiences perceived and felt 'now' rather than those remembered or anticipated. The emotion related to the Lungs is sadness or grief.

Note: The Triple Heater, unlike the other Zangfu Organs, is an 'Organ' which relates to no particular anatomical structure. It is easiest to consider it a catalyst for the functions of all the other Organs.

The following format explains the Organs and their functions together.

## The Kidneys

The Kidneys store Ki as 'Essence', which governs birth, growth and reproduction. In particular, the Essence controls bones, teeth, the brain, the spinal cord and nerves. (This is expressed as 'producing Marrow' in Oriental medicine). The Essence also enables the ears to function, and the hair to remain healthy and abundant.

Because the Kidney Essence is necessary for reproduction, the Kidneys give us the 'drive' to procreate, plus the willpower and instinct for survival.

The Kidneys provide the Ki to transform fluids into urine, and to control the flow of urine. As such they are said to govern water. They also influence defecation because they control the opening and closing of the anus as well as the urethra (i.e. the two lower orifices).

Another effect the Kidneys have upon Ki is to 'anchor' the Ki extracted from the air, sent down to them from the Lungs (expressed as 'controlling the reception of Ki').

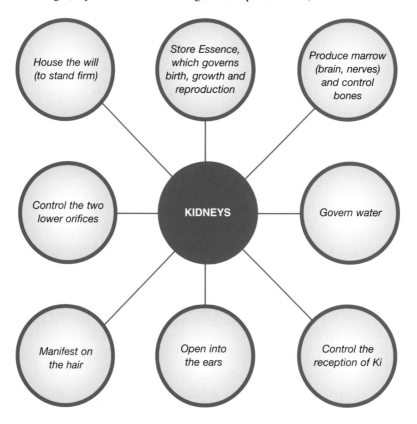

## The Bladder

The Bladder is intimately involved with the Kidneys in transforming fluids into urine. It then stores urine and in due course excretes it from the body.

As you can see, the Bladder as a Zangfu Organ has a relatively simple function. However, the Bladder channel runs parallel to the vertebral column, in very close proximity to the roots of both the peripheral nerves and the autonomic nervous system, thereby having a strong influence upon them.

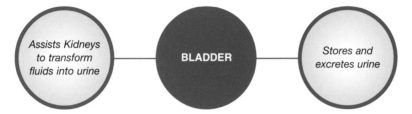

## The Liver

The Liver ensures that Ki flows smoothly through the body. In addition it stores much of the Blood during rest, and releases it during physical activity, ensuring the nourishment of the body, especially the joints, sinews, eyes, and nails.

In the mental sphere, the Liver is said to house the Ethereal Soul, which is our capacity for vision and planning. Unclear vision leads to bad planning, and can result in anger, the emotion associated with the Liver.

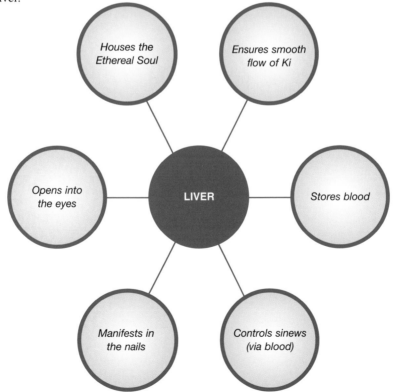

## The Gallbladder

The Gallbladder is very closely related to the Liver in function, in that it helps the Liver smooth the flow of Ki. Also, whilst the Liver is nourishing the joints, tendons and ligaments with Blood, the Gallbladder supplies them with Ki. As a physical structure, the Gallbladder stores and excretes bile.

Psychologically, the Gallbladder complements the Liver's 'plans' by giving the courage and initiative to make decisions. All plans are based upon multiple decisions.

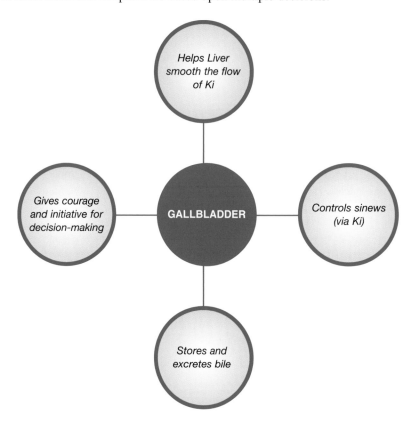

**The Heart**

The Heart governs the Blood by giving it impetus to circulate around the body. As part of this function it ensures the health and strength of the blood vessels. Furthermore, by controlling sweating, it regulates the viscosity of Blood through adjusting the amount of Body Fluids within it. A healthy Heart giving good circulation ultimately means a lustrous complexion.

The tongue, which commands a very rich supply of blood, is controlled mainly by the Heart. The Heart therefore controls the sense of taste and affects speech.

Finally, it is the Heart which has the most general influences on the Mind, governing mental activity, emotions, consciousness, thinking and sleep. Most of the other Organs influence specific nuances of the Mind, but it is the Heart and Blood which 'anchor' the Mind.

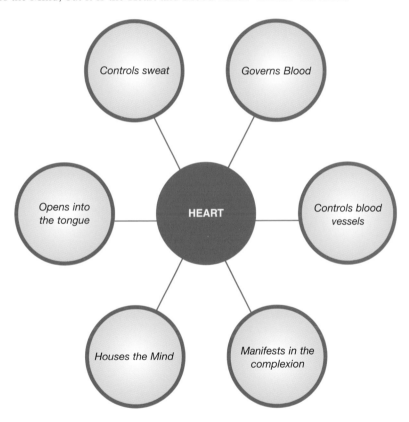

## The Small Intestine

The Small Intestine receives food and drink from the Stomach, and separates the nutritious part from the waste component. This process of selection or discrimination is mirrored on the mental level insofar as the Small Intestine gives the clarity of mind to make decisions. These functions are usually expressed as 'controls receiving and transforming' or 'separates the pure from the impure'.

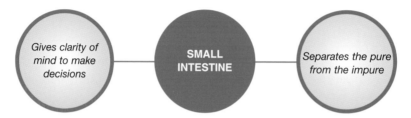

## The Heart Protector

The Heart Protector is closely related to the Heart. It relates to the pericardium, which is the outer covering of the heart organ. It acts like a bodyguard, protecting the Heart from invasion by pathogens, temperature changes and emotional trauma.

The Heart Protector also aids the Heart in governing the Blood and housing the Mind. Psychologically, the Heart energy influences one's relationship with oneself, whereas the Heart Protector influences the way we relate to others, especially in the close relationships.

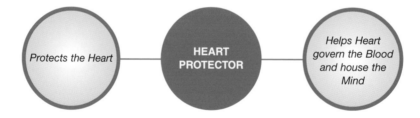

**The Triple Heater**

The Triple Heater is the only 'Organ' which does not equate with a physical organ. Its function is that of a catalyst regulating the functions of Organs in three distinct areas of the body. The thorax is known as the Upper Heater, which gives impetus to the Lung's function of distributing Body Fluids. The Middle Heater is between the diaphragm and the navel, facilitating digestion and the transporting of nutrients. The Lower Heater is the area below the navel, assisting the separation and excretion of fluids. The Triple Heater is therefore concerned with regulating the free passage of Body Fluids between these three regions.

The Triple Heater also distributes the strength of 'Ki' generated by the Hara (belly) to the Organs, and the periphery of the body, thereby helping to protect the body (by contributing to the Defensive Ki). It also helps to warm and protect the physical organs.

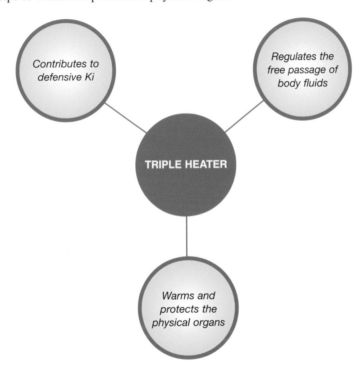

## The Spleen

The Spleen extracts Ki from food, sending some to the Lungs for combining with that extracted from air, to be circulated throughout the body by the Lungs. The Spleen also sends some Food-Ki to the Heart to enrich the Blood and give it impetus.

The Blood itself is transformed from ingested food and drink by the Spleen. The Spleen also 'controls' Blood by keeping it in the blood vessels.

The Spleen also separates the 'clean' part of ingested fluids from the 'dirty' part. The 'clean' part goes to the Lungs for distribution to the skin. The 'dirty' part goes to the Small Intestines for further refinement.

The Spleen ensures the strength and development of muscles by extracting nourishment from food and transporting it to the muscles and all other body parts; especially the limbs. It is because food passes the lips in the first stage of digestion that the lips are closely related to the Spleen, as is the mouth and therefore taste.

These functions basically mean 'digestion', traditionally expressed as 'governing transformation and transportation' (of food and fluids).

The Spleen is also responsible for preventing prolapses by 'holding up' organs and other body parts (expressed as 'raising Ki'). In the mental sphere, the Spleen influences thinking, analysing, concentrating and studying, thus ensuring strong powers of reasoning and memory.

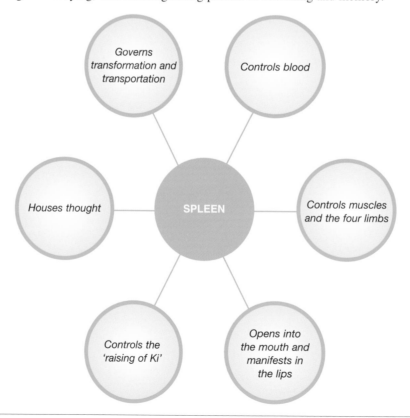

**The Stomach**

Through a process akin to fermentation ('rotting and ripening') the Stomach prepares ingested food for Ki extraction by the Spleen. It also helps the Spleen extract fluids from food to make Body Fluids.

Along with the Spleen, the Stomach also controls the transportation of food essences to the entire body, particularly the muscles and limbs.

It is the Ki of the Stomach which ensures that food is sent down to the Small Intestines, rather than 'rebelling' upwards to cause belching, hiccups and vomiting (expressed as 'controls descending Ki').

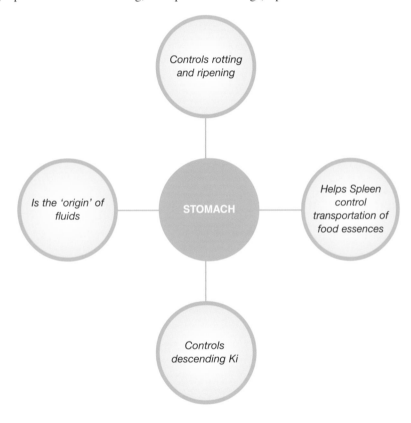

**The Lungs**

The Lungs extract Ki from air, which combines with Ki from food. They subsequently send this Ki through the Channels (and help the Heart to send Ki through the blood vessels) to energize all the physiological processes of the body. The Lungs also disperse Ki under the skin to provide the body's outer defensive layer, which protects us from pathogenic organisms, and extreme weather conditions such as cold.

In addition, the Lungs send Ki downwards to the Kidneys.

The Lungs also spread Body Fluids to the skin and body hair, moistening them and controlling the opening and closing of the pores, thereby influencing sweating. They also help the Bladder excrete urine, thus regulating the water passages.

Because the nose is the gateway of the breath, the nose, and therefore smell, is controlled by the Lungs.

The Lungs house the corporeal soul, which enables us to feel sensations and 'reality' by allowing us to experience 'now'.

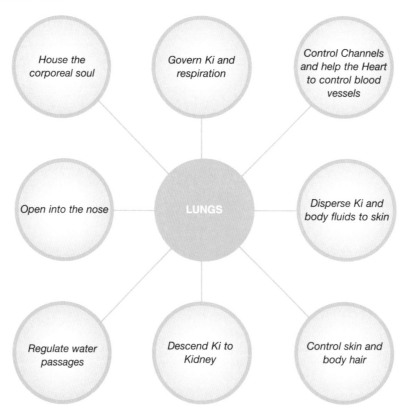

## The Large Intestine

The function of the Large Intestine is to receive the residue of food and drink from the Small Intestine, re-absorb some of the fluids, and excrete the remains as stools. In addition it has a role in the activity of defensive Ki, therefore influencing the body's immune system.

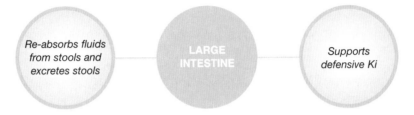

## The Chinese Channel Clock Cycle

The twelve primary channels are all linked together in one continuous loop; so if you could pull them out, unravel them and lay them on the ground, you would get a huge unbroken circle. Ki flows continuously around the loop, peaking in each channel and its respective Zang or Fu Organ in turn for a two-hour period. This causes each channel to be particularly active for the same period each day. This does not mean the channel is necessarily more jitsu during that time; this is more akin to an underlying wave of Ki. Having said that, a chronically jitsu channel will tend to be more blocked or hyperactive with Ki during its 'peak' time.

Doing shiatsu on or to a channel during its Ki peak is most effective, although not particularly convenient if the peak happens to be at 3 am to 5 am. However, it is also effective to address the channel when it is furthest from its Ki peak, which is twelve hours later.

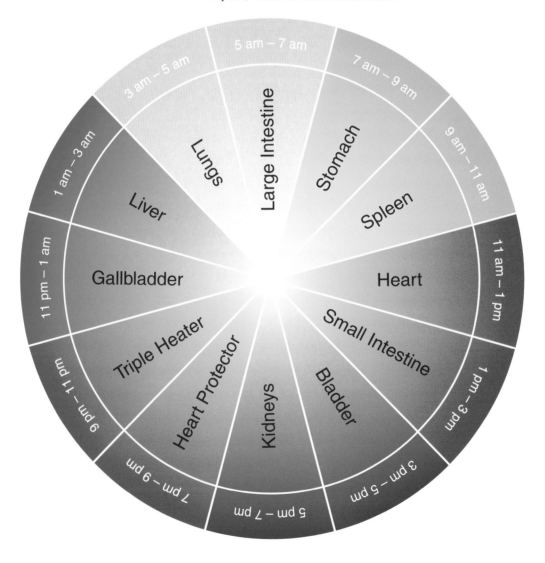

## Channels and Points

The *channels*, also known as *meridians*, are the pathways through the body along which Ki flows. For the level of shiatsu practice outlined in this book, we need to know about twelve major channels, each linked to the function of a particular organ, plus two extra channels that run up the midline of the torso and head on the front and back. The channel pathways run in a circuitous route through and around the body. They rise at intervals onto the surface, to give us the surface pathways as depicted in this chapter, and dip into the body to connect with the internal organs.

In the same way that arteries sub-divide into arterioles, which in turn sub-divide into capillaries, the major or 'classical' channels have extensions to their distribution and wider connections with other minor channels to create a network over and throughout the body. In fact, all parts of the body are touched by Ki, brought to them by the channels via their sub-divisions and branches. The detailed location of minor channels and channel extensions are not relevant to the contents of this book and are thus not shown.

Each major channel is paired with another channel. In general, the channels, which exist more on the front of the body, are Yin channels, as they relate to Yin organs and because the front of the body is more Yin than the back (see Yin-Yang theory, pages 130–133). Conversely, the channels, which exist on the back of the body, are Yang channels as they relate to Yang organs and because the back of the body is more Yang than the front.

There are twelve channels that mirror themselves bilaterally on the body meaning that the channel map for the left half of the body is a mirror image of the right side of the body. The Conception Vessel (Ren) and Governing Vessel (Du) are single pathways because they circulate the midline of the head and torso.

Note: The location of tsubos along the channels, are frequently measured in multiples of *cun*. A *cun* is a unit of measurement used in Oriental medicine that is approximately equivalent to the recipient's thumb at its widest part.

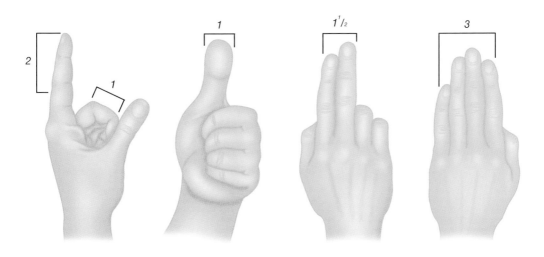

# The Lung Channel

### Lu-1 Central Treasury

Below the lateral extremity of the clavicle, approximately 1 cun inferior and slightly lateral to Lu-2, and approximately 6 cun lateral to the anterior midline. Locate with the patient's arm stretched forward (flexion of the shoulder).
*Main Areas it Benefits:* Chest. Lungs. Nose. Shoulder.
*Main Functions:* Benefits respiration. Regulates chest qi. Releases the exterior. Clears heat. Tonifies Lung qi.

### Lu-2 Cloud Gate

At the centre of the depression of the delto-pectoral triangle, below the lateral extremity of the clavicle, approximately 6 cun lateral to the anterior midline Locate with the patient's shoulder in flexion (arm stretched out forward).
*Main Areas it Benefits:* Shoulder. Arms. Chest. Lungs.
*Main Functions:* Regulates qi. Alleviates pain.

### Lu-5 Cubit Marsh

On the cubital crease in the depression on the radial side of the tendon of biceps brachii muscle. Locate with the elbow flexed.
*Main Areas it Benefits:* Lungs. Chest. Elbow. Upper Jiao.
*Main Functions:* Dispels phlegm. Opens the water passages. Alleviates cough. Clears the Lungs.

### Lu-6 Collection Hole

On the anterior aspect of the forearm, 7 cun above Lu-9, on the line joining Lu-5 and Lu-9. To aid location, Lu-6 is 1 cun above the midpoint of the line connecting Lu-5 with Lu-9.
*Main Areas it Benefits:* Nose. Lungs. Skin. Forearm.
*Main Functions:* Releases the exterior. Induces sweating. Clears heat from the upper Jiao. Arrests bleeding.

### Lu-7 Interrupted Sequence

On the lateral aspect of the radius, at the base of the styloid process, 1.5 cun proximal to the transverse wrist crease. In the narrow 'V' shaped crevice, between the tendons of brachioradialis and abductor pollicis longus. To aid location, slide the tip of the index finger proximally up from LI-5, to slip into the shallow crevice.
*Main Areas it Benefits:* Head. Face. Back of neck. Nose. Throat. Lungs. Chest. Bladder. Forearm.
*Main Functions:* Descends and disperses Lung qi. Releases the exterior. Opens the Ren Mai. Nourishes yin and moistens fluids. Augments Lung qi.

### Lu-9 Great Abyss

On the transverse wrist crease, in the depression on the radial (lateral) side of the radial artery. Lateral to the tendon of flexor carpi radialis and medial to the tendon of abductor pollicis longus.
*Main Areas it Benefits:* Chest. Lungs. Blood vessels.
*Main Functions:* Tonifies chest qi. Strengthens the breath and voice. Nourishes Lung yin. Transforms phlegm. Benefits the vessels and improves circulation.

### Lu-10 Fish Border

On the thenar eminence, halfway along the first metacarpal bone at the border of the red and white skin (the junction of the skin or the palmar and dorsal surfaces), between the flesh and bone.
*Main Areas it Benefits:* Lungs. Throat. Thumb.
*Main Functions:* Clears exterior heat and phlegm and fire toxins. Benefits the throat.

### Lu-11 Lesser Metal

On the radial (lateral) side of the thumb, approximately 0.1 cun proximal to the corner of the nail. At the intersection of two lines following the radial border of the nail and the base of the nail.
*Main Areas it Benefits:* Throat. Lung channel. Mind.
*Main Functions:* Dispels exterior heat and wind. Restores consciousness.

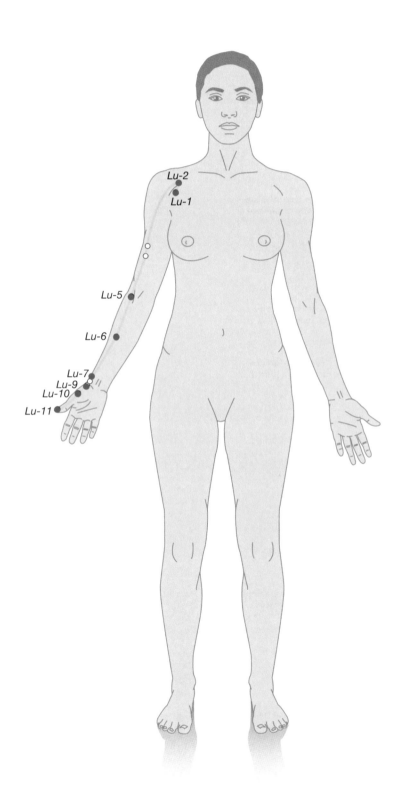

# The Large Intestine Channel

### LI-1 Metal Yang

On the radial (lateral) side of the index finger, approximately 0.1 cun proximal to the corner of the base of the nail.
*Main Areas it Benefits:* Throat. Large Intestine channel. Mind.
*Main Functions:* Restores consciousness. Benefits the throat.

### LI-4 Uniting Valley

Between the first and second metacarpal bones close to the radial border of the midpoint of the second metacarpal bone. To aid location, it is at the highest point of the bulge of the dorsal interosseous muscle when the thumb is adducted. Alternatively, it can be located at the end of the crease formed between the index finger and thumb, when the thumb is adducted.
*Main Areas it Benefits:* Hand. Face. Sense organs. Mouth. Teeth. Eyes. Nose. Chest. Throat. Mind. Lungs. Abdomen. Intestine.
*Main Functions:* Analgesia point. Moves stuck qi. Dissipates fullness and releases pathogens.

### LI-5 Yang Stream

On the lateral aspect of the wrist, at the centre of the depression known as the anatomical snuffbox formed by the tendons of the extensor pollicis longus and brevis muscles, between the scaphoid and radius. To aid location, extend the thumb to define the anatomical snuffbox.
*Main Areas it Benefits:* Wrist. Hand.
*Main Functions:* Alleviates pain and swelling.

### LI-10 Arm Three Miles

On the radial side of the dorsal surface of the forearm on the line connecting LI-5 and LI-11, 2 cun distal to the cubital crease and LI-11. Locate with the elbow flexed to 90°.
*Main Areas it Benefits:* Forearm. Arm. Shoulder. Stomach. Intestines.
*Main Functions:* Strengthens the arms. Alleviates pain.

### LI-11 Pond at the Bend

At the lateral end of the cubital crease when the elbow is flexed. Approximately midway between Lu-5 and the lateral epicondyle of the humerus.
*Main Areas it Benefits:* Elbow. Forearm. Throat. Face (nose, eyes, mouth, ears). Lungs. Abdomen. Intestines.
*Main Functions:* Clears heat and damp-heat. Regulates qi. Dispels stasis.

### LI-15 Shoulder Bone

In the depression anterior and inferior to the acromion when the arm is abducted. Locate LI-15 directly anterior to SJ-14.
*Main Area it Benefits:* Shoulder.
*Main Functions:* Regulates qi and Blood. Dispels stasis. Alleviates pain.

### LI-16 Great Bone

On the superior aspect of the shoulder, at the centre of the large depression medial to the acromion process, formed by the acromial (lateral) extremity of the clavicle and the scapular spine. In the trapezius and supraspinatus muscles.
*Main Area it Benefits:* Shoulder.
*Main Functions:* Regulates qi and Blood. Dispels stasis. Opens the chest. Alleviates pain.

### LI-18 Three Cun Prominence

Between the two heads of the sternocleidomastoid muscle, directly lateral to St-9, level with the tip of the laryngeal prominence (Adam's Apple).
*Main Area it Benefits:* Throat.
*Main Functions:* Alleviates swelling and pain.

### LI-20 Receiving Fragrance

In the nasolabial sulcus, level with the midpoint of the lateral border of the ala nasi.
*Main Area it Benefits:* Nose.
*Main Functions:* Improves breathing and smell. Clears heat and wind.

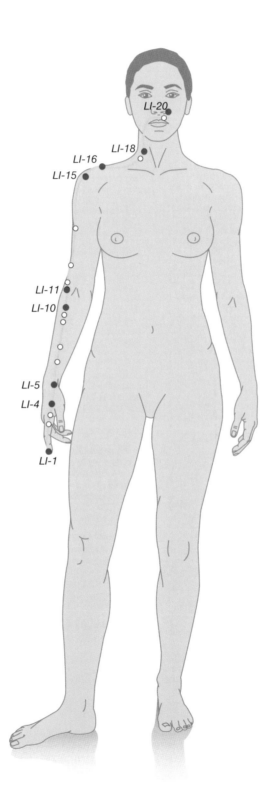

LI-20

LI-18

LI-16

LI-15

LI-11

LI-10

LI-5

LI-4

LI-1

# The Stomach Channel

### St-1 Tear Container

Between the eyeball and the midpoint of the infraorbital ridge, level with the centre of the pupil when the eye is focused straight ahead.
*Main Area it Benefits:* Eyes and area below.
*Main Functions:* Benefits the eyes and area below. Improves vision. Dispels wind and clears heat.

### St-3 Great Bone Hole

Below the zygomatic arch, directly below St-1 and St-2, approximately level with the lower border of the ala nasi.
*Main Areas it Benefits:* Cheeks and centre of the face. Nose. Sinuses. Eyes. Gums and teeth.
*Main Functions:* Dispels wind and clears heat. Opens the nose. Alleviates pain.

### St-9 Man's Prognosis

In the carotid triangle, anterior to the border of the sternocleidomastoid muscle, between the common carotid artery and thyroid cartilage, approximately 1.5 cun lateral to the tip of the laryngeal prominence (Adam's Apple).
*Main Areas it Benefits:* Throat. Thyroid gland. Face. Head. Brain. Heart. Blood vessels.
*Main Functions:* Descends rising yang. Clears heat. Calms the mind and body. Increases parasympathetic nervous system activity. Lowers heart rate and output. Benefits the throat and thyroid.

### St-18 Breast Root

In the fifth intercostal space directly below the nipple (if there is minimal breast tissue), 4 cun lateral to the anterior midline (approximately level with Kd-22).
*Main Areas it Benefits:* Breasts. Lungs. Liver and chest.
*Main Functions:* Dispels stasis. Benefits the breast.

### St-25 Celestial Pivot

2 cun lateral to the centre of the umbilicus (Ren-8), on the rectus abdominis muscle.
*Main Areas it Benefits:* Intestines. Umbilicus. Abdomen. Uterus.
*Main Functions:* Clears dampness and Heat. Regulates qi in the lower Jiao. Benefits the intestines.

### St-30 Qi Surge

2 cun lateral to the anterior midline (Ren-2), superior and slightly lateral to the pubic tubercle, on the medial side of the femoral artery and vein.
*Main Areas it Benefits:* Reproductive organs. Uterus. Testicles. Bladder. Intestines. Lower abdomen.
*Main Functions:* Benefits the lower Jiao. Regulates menstruation. Improves sexual function and fertility.

### St-34 Ridge Mound

In the depression 2 cun (one patella's length) proximal to the latero-superior border of the patella, on the line connecting the anterior superior iliac spine to the lateral border of the patella.
*Main Areas it Benefits:* Stomach. Epigastrium. Lower Limbs. Knees.
*Main Functions:* Pacifies the Stomach. Descends rebellious Ki. Benefits the knees.

### St-35 Calf's Nose

Lateral to the patellar tendon, in the depression appearing when the knee is flexed. In the knee joint space directly below the patella. This point is also called the lateral eye of the knee.
*Main Area it Benefits:* Knees.
*Main Functions:* Alleviates pain, stiffness and swelling. Strengthens the knees.

### St-36 Leg Three Miles

One finger width lateral to the tibial crest, level with the lower border of the tibial tuberosity. 3 cun below the large depression lateral to the patellar tendon when the knee is flexed (St-35). Approximately 1 cun anterior and inferior to GB-34.
*Main Areas it Benefits:* Stomach. Digestive system. Abdomen. Chest. Lower limb. Knee. Whole body.
*Main Functions:* Tonifies qi, Blood, fluids, yin and yang. Boosts the Stomach and Spleen. Benefits the abdomen and chest.

### St-40 Abundant Bulge

On the lower leg, 8 cun below the knee crease, two finger widths lateral to the St-35 and the lateral malleolus. To aid location, it is halfway between the St-35 and the lateral malleolus.
*Main Areas it Benefits:* Chest. Head. Mind. Lungs. Stomach. Heart.
*Main Functions:* Resolves phlegm and transforms damp. Opens the chest. Relieves cough. Calms and clears the mind. Benefits the digestive system.

### St-41 Dividing Cleft

On the anterior aspect of the ankle, level of the tip of the lateral malleolus (when the foot is flexed at right angles), in a depression between the tendons of extensor digitorum longus and hallucis longus muscles.
*Main Areas it Benefits:* Ankle. Foot. Stomach. Head.
*Main Functions:* Alleviates pain. Clears heat.

### St-42 Surging Yang

1.3 cun distal to St-41 at the high point of the dorsum of the foot in the depression formed by the second and third metatarsal bones and the cuneiform bones, where the pulse of the dorsalis pedis artery can be felt.
*Main Areas it Benefits:* Stomach. Middle Jiao. Foot. Mind.
*Main Functions:* Tonifies qi and yang.

### St-44 Inner Court

Between the second and third toes, proximal to the margin of the web (at the end of the crease), between the metatarsophalangeal joints.
*Main Areas it Benefits:* Stomach. Digestive system. Face. Mouth. Eyes. Head.
*Main Function:* Clears heat.

### St-45 Running Point

0.1 cun proximal to the lateral corner of the base of the second toenail.
*Main Areas it Benefits:* Face. Eyes. Mouth. Stomach. Stomach channel. Mind.
*Main Function:* Resuscitates consciousness.

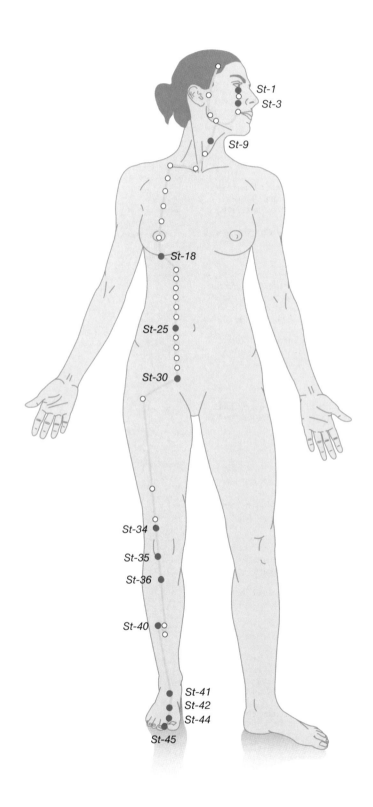

# The Spleen Channel

### Sp-1 Hidden White
0.1 cun proximal to the medial corner of the base of the big toenail.
*Main Areas it Benefits:* Uterus. Blood vessels. Mind.
*Main Functions:* Arrests bleeding. Lifts qi. Calms and clears the mind.

### Sp-3 Supreme White
On the medial aspect of the foot, in the small depression proximal and inferior to the head of the first metatarsal bone on the junction of the skin of the plantar and dorsal surface.
*Main Areas it Benefits:* Digestive system. Intestines. Urinary system. Muscles. Mind.
*Main Functions:* Transforms dampness. Tonifies Spleen qi and yang.

### Sp-4 Grandfather Grandson
On the medial aspect of the foot, in the depression distal and inferior to the base of the first metatarsal bone, at the junction of the skin of the plantar and dorsal surface. Locate by sliding your fingertip about 1 cun proximally from Sp-3 along the shaft of the first metatarsal, into the depression at the base of the bone.
*Main Areas it Benefits:* The three Jiao. Stomach. Abdomen. Uterus. Heart. Mind.
*Main Functions:* Opens the Chong Mai. Regulates qi. Dispels Blood stasis. Benefits menstruation.

### Sp-6 Three Yin Intersection
3 cun superior to the prominence of the medial malleolus, posterior to the medial tibial border. To aid location, Sp-6 is approximately one hand width proximal to the medial malleolus.
*Main Areas it Benefits:* Entire body, particularly abdomen. Liver. Spleen. Kidney.
*Main Functions:* Boosts the Spleen and Stomach. Transforms dampness. Nourishes Blood and yin. Calms the mind. Regulates qi and Blood. Benefits menstruation. Promotes labour.

### Sp-8 Earth's Cure
5 cun inferior to the knee crease, in the depression posterior to the medial tibial border. Between the soleus muscle and the tibia. To aid location, Sp-8 is one third of the way between the popliteal (knee) crease and the prominence of the medial malleolus, or 3 cun (one hand width) distal to Sp-9.
*Main Areas it Benefits:* Uterus. Abdomen. Knee.
*Main Functions:* Invigorates Blood. Dispels stasis. Regulates menstruation.

### Sp-9 Yin Mound Spring
In the depression below the medial tibial condyle, between the tibial border and the gastrocnemius muscle. Locate with the knee flexed.
*Main Areas it Benefits:* Lower Jiao. Urogenital system. Intestines. Abdomen. Knee.
*Main Functions:* Drains dampness. Regulates the lower Jiao.

### Sp-10 Sea of Blood
In the depression on the protuberance of the vastus medialis muscle, 2 cun (one patella length) proximal to the medial superior border of the patella. Directly above Sp-9 and level with St-34. Locate and treat with the knee flexed.
*Main Areas it Benefits:* Skin. Gynaecological system. Genitals.
*Main Functions:* Invigorates and cools Blood.

### Sp-15 Great Horizontal
In the depression on the lateral border of the rectus abdominis muscle, 4 cun lateral to the centre of the umbilicus.
*Main Areas it Benefits:* Intestines. Abdomen.
*Main Functions:* Tonifies the Spleen. Regulates the intestines and treats constipation.

### Sp-20 Complete Nourishment
On the chest, one intercostal space below Lu-1. Approximately 6 cun lateral to the anterior midline.
*Main Areas it Benefits:* Chest. Ribs. Breast.
*Main Functions:* Regulates qi and Blood.

### Sp-21 Great Embrace
On the mid axillary line, midway between the centre of the axilla and the lower border of the eleventh rib. Sp-21 usually falls in the seventh intercostal space, but in some cases it may be in the sixth. To aid location, it is approximately one hand's width below the axilla.
*Main Areas it Benefits:* Ribs. Thorax. Breast.
*Main Functions:* Invigorates Blood. Warms. Dispels stasis.

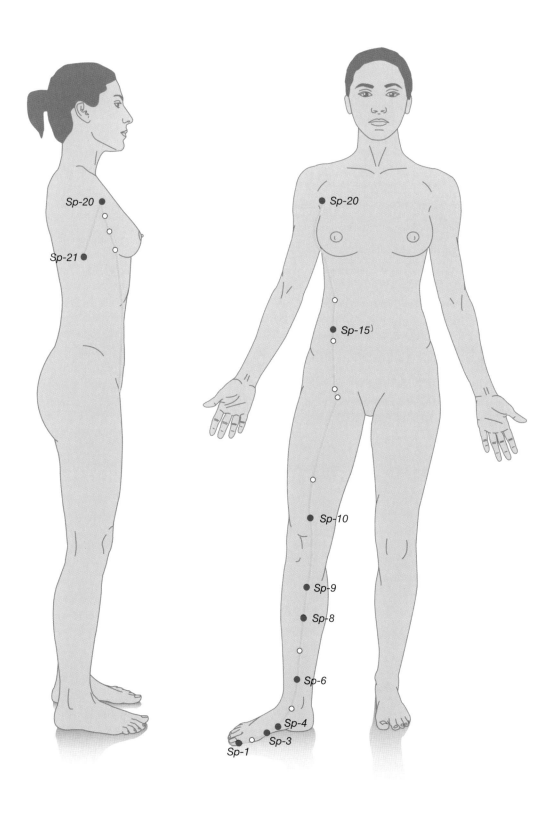

Sp-20

Sp-21

Sp-20

Sp-15

Sp-10

Sp-9

Sp-8

Sp-6

Sp-4

Sp-3

Sp-1

# The Heart Channel

### He-1 Highest Spring

At the centre of the axilla, medial to the axillary artery. Locate and treat with the arm lifted above the head. To aid location palpate the lateral inferior border of the pectoralis major muscle.

*Main Areas it Benefits:* Axilla. Shoulder. Chest. Heart.

*Main Functions:* Clears heat. Regulates Sweat. Regulates Heart qi.

### He-3 Lesser Sea

In the depression anterior to the medial epicondyle of the humerus near the medial end of the transverse cubital crease when the elbow is fully flexed. To aid location, it is approximately one finger width diagonally anterior to the tip of the epicondyle.

*Main Areas it Benefits:* Elbow. Chest. Heart.

*Main Functions:* Clears heat. Transforms phlegm. Soothes the heart.

### He-5 Inward Connection

On the radial side of the tendon of flexor carpi ulnaris, 1 cun proximal to He-7.

*Main Areas it Benefits:* Wrist. Heart. Tongue. Bladder.

*Main Functions:* Regulates and tonifies Heart qi. Calms the mind. Benefits the tongue. Regulates speech.

### He-6 Yin Cleft

On the radial side of the tendon of flexor carpi ulnaris, 0.5 cun proximal to He-7.

*Main Areas it Benefits:* Exterior. Heart. Mind. Wrist.

*Main Functions:* Clears heat and fire. Calms the mind. Secures sweat.

### He-7 Spirit Gate

At the wrist joint, in the depression on the radial side of the tendon of flexor carpi ulnaris. To aid location, He-7 is level with the proximal border of the pisiform bone when the wrist is flexed. This usually falls on the distal wrist crease.

*Main Areas it Benefits:* Heart. Mind. Wrist.

*Main Functions:* Calms the mind. Nourishes Heart Blood. Soothes the Heart. Clears heat.

### He-9 Lesser Surge

On the radial side of the dorsal aspect of the little finger, 0.1 cun proximal to the corner of the base of the nail.

*Main Areas it Benefits:* Mind. Heart. Chest.

*Main Functions:* Resuscitates consciousness. Regulates Heart qi.

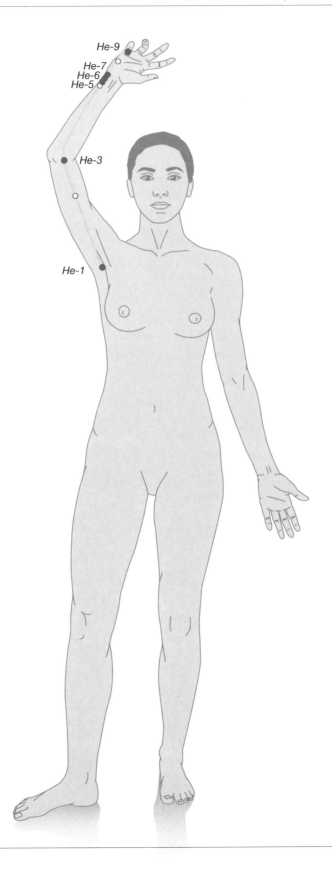

He-9
He-7
He-6
He-5
He-3
He-1

# The Small Intestine Channel

**SI-1 Lesser Marsh**

On the ulnar side of the little finger, 0.1 cun proximal to the corner of the base of the nail.
*Main Areas it Benefits:* Breast. Mind.
*Main Functions:* Promotes lactation. Restores consciousness. Releases the exterior.

**SI-3 Back Stream**

When a loose fist is formed, at the ulnar end of the distal transverse palmar crease, in the depression proximal to the head of the fifth metacarpal bone.
*Main Areas it Benefits:* Hand. Neck. Spine. Sense organs. Mind. Brain. Nervous system. Heart.
*Main Functions:* Descends yang. Clears heat. Opens the Du Mai. Benefits the spine.

**SI-4 Wrist Bone**

On the ulnar border of the hand, in the depression between the base of the fifth metacarpal and the triquetral bone. Locate with the hand in a loose fist.
*Main Areas it Benefits:* Wrist. Hand.
*Main Functions:* Alleviates swelling and pain anywhere along the channel.

**SI-8 Small Sea**

In the depression between the olecranon of the ulna and the medial epicondyle of the humerus. Locate with the elbow flexed.
*Main Areas it Benefits:* Elbow. Forearm.
*Main Functions:* Regulates qi and Blood. Alleviates pain.

**SI-10 Upper Arm Shu**

Above the end of the posterior axillary fold when the arm is adducted, in the depression below the lower border of the spine of the scapula.
*Main Areas it Benefits:* Shoulder. Scapula. Arm.
*Main Functions:* Regulates qi and Blood. Alleviates pain.

**SI-11 Heavenly Gathering**

In the tender depression at the centre of the scapula, midway between its medial and lateral border, one-third of the distance along the line joining the midpoint of the lower border of the scapular spine to the inferior angle of scapula.
*Main Areas it Benefits:* Scapula. Supraspinatus muscle.
*Main Functions:* Regulates qi and Blood. Alleviates pain.

**SI-17 Heavenly Appearance**

In the depression immediately posterior to the angle of the mandible, at the anterior border of the sternocleidomastoid muscle.
*Main Areas it Benefits:* Throat. Ears.
*Main Functions:* Regulates qi and Blood. Alleviates pain. Relieves swelling.

**SI-18 Cheek Bone Crevice**

Directly below the outer canthus of the eye, in the depression at the lower border of the zygomatic arch.
*Main Areas it Benefits:* Throat. Ears.
*Main Functions:* Regulates qi and Blood. Alleviates pain. Relieves swelling.

**SI-19 Palace of Hearing**

Anterior to the tragus of the ear in the depression formed when the mouth is opened.
*Main Areas it Benefits:* Temple. Jaw. Ears.
*Main Functions:* Regulates qi and Blood. Alleviates pain. Clears heat. Improves hearing.

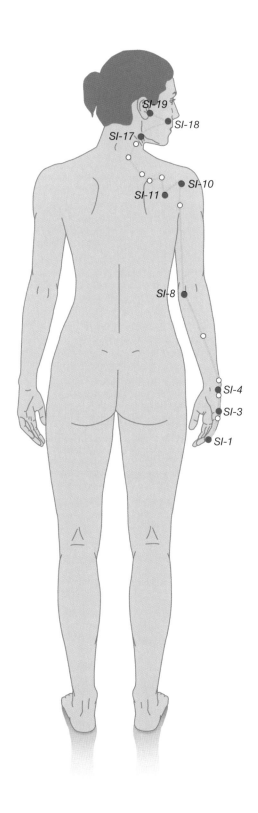

# The Bladder Channel

### Bl-1 Bright Eyes

Approximately 0.1 cun medial and superior to the inner canthus of the eye. Locate and treat with the eyes closed.
*Main Area it Benefits:* Eyes.
*Main Functions:* Clears and brightens the eyes. Improves vision. Dispels wind and clears heat. Alleviates pain. Nourishes yin.

### Bl-2 Gathered Bamboo

Near the medial end of the eyebrow, in a small depression superior to the inner canthus and Bl-1.
*Main Areas it Benefits:* Eyes. Forehead.
*Main Functions:* Regulates qi and Blood. Alleviates pain. Dispels wind. Clears heat.

### Bl-10 Celestial Pillar

On the nape of the neck, in the depression of the lateral border of the trapezius muscle, 1.3 cun lateral to the midpoint of the posterior hairline (Du-15).
*Main Areas it Benefits:* Neck. Head. Upper back.
*Main Functions:* Dispels wind and cold. Regulates qi and Blood. Calms the mind.
*Note:* All the points on the inner Bladder channel line on the back (Bl-11 to Bl-25) are located at the highest part of the erector spinae muscle group, 1.5 cun lateral to the posterior midline.

### Bl-11 Great Shuttle

1.5 cun lateral to the lower border of the spinous process of T1.
*Main Areas it Benefits:* Lungs. Chest. Exterior.
*Main Functions:* Dispels wind and cold. Regulates Lung qi.

### Bl-13 Lung Shu

1.5 cun lateral to the lower border of the spinous process of T3.
*Main Areas it Benefits:* Lungs. Chest. Exterior.
*Main Functions:* Tonifies and regulates Lung qi. Releases the exterior. Nourishes yin.

### Bl-14 Absolute Yin Shu

1.5 cun lateral to the lower border of the spinous process of T4.
*Main Areas it Benefits:* Chest. Heart.
*Main Functions:* Regulates chest qi. Benefits the Heart and Liver.

### Bl-15 Heart Shu

1.5 cun lateral to the lower border of the spinous process of T5.
*Main Areas it Benefits:* Chest. Heart.
*Main Functions:* Regulates qi and Blood in the chest. Tonifies Heart qi. Calms the mind.

### Bl-17 Diaphragm Shu

1.5 cun lateral to the lower border of the spinous process of T7.
*Main Areas it Benefits:* Diaphragm. Chest. Abdomen.
*Main Functions:* Nourishes and invigorates Blood. Clears Blood heat. Relaxes the diaphragm. Benefits the skin.

### Bl-18 Liver Shu

1.5 cun lateral to the lower border of the spinous process of T9.
*Main Areas it Benefits:* Liver. Hypochondrium. Abdomen. Eyes.
*Main Functions:* Spreads Liver qi. Dispels stasis. Nourishes Blood. Clears heat and dampness. Benefits the eyes.

### Bl-19 Gallbladder Shu

1.5 cun lateral to the lower border of the spinous process of T10.
*Main Areas it Benefits:* Gallbladder. Liver. Hypochondrium. Abdomen.
*Main Functions:* Spreads Gallbladder and Liver qi. Dispels stasis. Alleviates pain. Clears dampness and heat.

### Bl-20 Spleen Shu

1.5 cun lateral to the lower border of the spinous process of T11.
*Main Areas it Benefits:* Spleen. Stomach. Intestines. Digestive system. Muscles. Entire body.
*Main Functions:* Boosts Spleen and Stomach qi. Boosts transformation and movement. Clears dampness.

### Bl-21 Stomach Shu

1.5 cun lateral to the lower border of the spinous process of T12.
*Main Areas it Benefits:* Digestive system. Stomach.
*Main Functions:* Regulates Stomach qi. Benefits the digestion. Descends rebellious qi.

### Bl-22 Sanjiao Shu

1.5 cun lateral to the lower border of the spinous process of L1.
*Main Area it Benefits:* Urinary system.
*Main Functions:* Resolves dampness. Opens the water passages. Harmonises Sanjiao.

### Bl-23 Kidney Shu

1.5 cun lateral to the lower border of the spinous process of L2.
*Main Areas it Benefits:* Kidneys. Lumbar area. Abdomen. Genitourinary system. Entire body.
*Main Functions:* Boosts the Kidneys. Tonifies yang and warms the lower Jiao. Nourishes yin and cools empty heat. Resolves dampness. Benefits urination. Alleviates pain.

### Bl-25 Large Intestine Shu

1.5 cun lateral to the lower border of the spinous process of L4.
*Main Areas it Benefits:* Intestines. Lumbar area.
*Main Functions:* Alleviates constipation and diarrhoea. Regulates qi and alleviates pain.

### Bl-27 Small Intestine Shu

On the sacrum at the level of the first posterior sacral foramen, 1.5 cun lateral to the posterior midline.
*Main Areas it Benefits:* Small Intestine. Sacroiliac joint. Urinary system.
*Main Functions:* Benefits the urinary system. Clears dampness and heat. Alleviates pain.

### Bl-28 Bladder Shu

On the sacrum at the level of the second posterior sacral foramen, 1.5 cun lateral to the posterior midline.
*Main Areas it Benefits:* Bladder. Sacroiliac joint. Urinary system.
*Main Functions:* Regulates the Bladder. Benefits the urinary system. Clears dampness and heat. Alleviates pain.

### Bl-36 Support

At the centre of the transverse gluteal crease, in a depression, inferior to the gluteus maximus, between the biceps femoris and semitendinosus muscles.
*Main Areas it Benefits:* Buttocks. Thigh. Lower limb.
*Main Functions:* Regulates qi and Blood. Alleviates pain and sciatica.

### Bl-40 Middle of the Crease

At the midpoint of the popliteal crease between the tendons of biceps femoris and semitendinosus muscles.
*Main Areas it Benefits:* Lower back. Knee. Lower limbs.
*Main Functions:* Regulates qi and Blood. Alleviates pain. Clears heat.

### Bl-43 Vital Region Shu

3 cun lateral to the lower border of the spinous process of T4, level with Bl-14. Just medial to the medial border of the scapula if the shoulder is relaxed.
*Main Areas it Benefits:* Chest. Lungs. Heart.
*Main Functions:* Regulates chest qi. Strengthens the Lungs and Heart.

## Bl-52 Willpower Room

3 cun lateral to the lower border of the spinous process of L2, level with Bl-23.
*Main Areas it Benefits:* Kidneys. Lumbar area. Lower Jiao.
*Main Functions:* Boosts the Kidneys and the Will.

## Bl-57 Mountain Support

Inferior to the belly of the gastrocnemius muscle between Bl-40 and Bl-60, in the depression formed when the heel is lifted.
*Main Areas it Benefits:* Anus. Calf and leg.
*Main Functions:* Regulates qi and Blood and alleviates pain. Treats haemorrhoids.

## Bl-60 Kunlun Mountains

In the depression between the tip of the lateral malleolus and the Achilles tendon.
*Main Areas it Benefits:* Lower limb. Ankle. Spine and neck. Head. Uterus.
*Main Functions:* Expels exterior pathogens. Descends rising yang. Subdues wind and clears heat. Regulates qi and Blood and dispels stasis from the lower Jiao. Promotes labour. Alleviates pain.

## Bl-67 Reaching Yin

0.1 cun proximal to the lateral corner of the fifth toenail.
*Main Areas it Benefits:* Uterus. Head.
*Main Functions:* Corrects position of foetus. Dispels exterior pathogens.

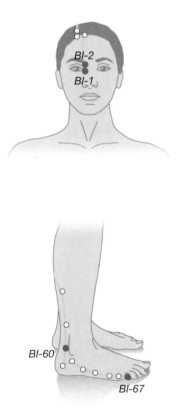

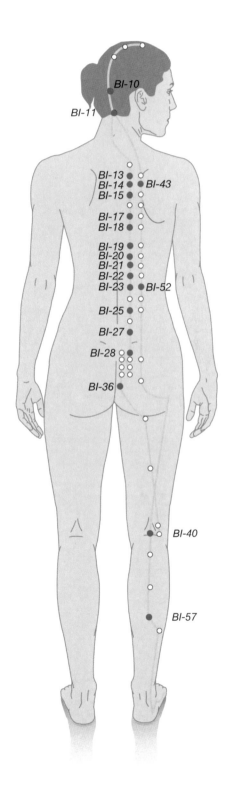

# The Kidney Channel

### Kd-1 Bubbling Spring

On the sole of the foot, in the visible depression formed when the foot is plantarflexed, between the second and third metatarsal bones, approximately one third of the distance from the base of the second toe to the heel.

*Main Areas it Benefits:* Head. Mind. Sole of the foot. Entire body.

*Main Functions:* Clears fire. Sedates interior wind. Calms the mind. Resuscitates consciousness.

### Kd-3 Supreme Stream

In the depression between the tip of the medial malleolus and the Achilles tendon when the foot is at right angles. Opposite and slightly superior to Bl-60.

*Main Areas it Benefits:* Kidneys. Spine. Entire body.

*Main Functions:* Augments Kidney yin and yang. Tonifies yuan qi. Benefits the genitourinary system. Increases fertility.

### Kd-6 Shining Sea

In the depression approximately 1 cun below the prominence of the medial malleolus.

*Main Areas it Benefits:* Head. Eyes. Ears. Throat. Mind. Lower Jiao. Uterus.

*Main Functions:* Nourishes yin. Cools empty heat.

### Kd-7 Returning Flow

2 cun proximal to Kd-3, in the depression anterior to the border of the Achilles tendon.

*Main Areas it Benefits:* Water passages. Lower Jiao.

*Main Functions:* Regulates sweat and urination. Reduces swelling. Tonifies Kidney yang.

### Kd-10 Yin Valley

At the medial end of the popliteal crease between the tendon of semitendinosus and the lower end of the semimembranosus muscle, located with the knee flexed.

*Main Areas it Benefits:* Lower Jiao. Genitourinary system.

*Main Functions:* Nourishes yin and cools lower Jiao heat. Transforms dampness.

### Kd-27 Spirit Residence

In the depression inferior to the medial end of the clavicle, 2 cun lateral to the midline (Ren-21).

*Main Areas it Benefits:* Chest. Throat.

*Main Functions:* Descends rebellious qi. Regulates qi.

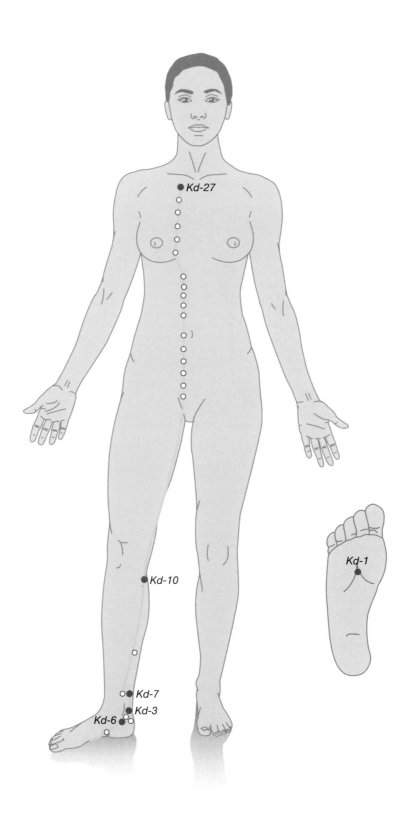

# The Heart Protector (Pericardium) Channel

### P-1 Heavenly Pool

Approximately 1 cun lateral and superior to the nipple, in the fourth intercostal space.
*Main Areas it Benefits:* Breast. Chest. Ribs. Heart.
*Main Functions:* Treats disorders of the breasts and chest.

### P-3 Marsh at the Bend

On the transverse cubital crease, in the depression on the medial (ulnar) side of the tendon of the biceps brachii muscle. Locate with the elbow slightly bent.
*Main Areas it Benefits:* Chest. Heart. Stomach. Elbow.
*Main Functions:* Clears heat. Dispels stasis. Descends rebellious qi.

### P-6 Inner Pass

2 cun proximal P-7 at the transverse wrist crease between the tendons on the palmaris longus and flexor carpi radialis muscles. If the palmaris longus is absent, locate P-6 on the ulnar side of the flexor carpi radialis tendon.
*Main Areas it Benefits:* Chest. Heart. Mind. Stomach. Wrist. Forearm. Neck.
*Main Functions:* Regulates qi and Blood. Dispels stasis. Relaxes the chest. Calms the mind. Descends rebellious qi. Harmonises the Stomach.

### P-7 Great Mound

On the wrist crease in the depression between the tendons of palmaris longus and flexor carpi radialis muscles. Approximately midway between He-7 and Lu-9.
*Main Areas it Benefits:* Wrist. Chest. Heart. Stomach.
*Main Functions:* Regulates qi and Blood. Relaxes the chest. Calms the mind. Descends rebellious qi.

### P-8 Palace of Toil

At the centre of the palm, in the depression between the second and third metacarpals, on the radial side of the third metacarpal. To aid location, if the fist is clenched, P-8 is where the tip of the middle finger touches the palm.
*Main Areas it Benefits:* Palm. Chest. Heart. Mind.
*Main Functions:* Clears heat. Restores consciousness. Calms the mind. Descends rebellious qi. Focuses qi in qigong therapy.

### P-9 Central Surge

At the centre of the tip of the middle finger. Alternatively, 0.1 cun proximal to the corner of the base of the nail on the radial side of the middle finger.
*Main Areas it Benefits:* Heart. Mind.
*Main Functions:* Restores consciousness. Opens the orifices. Opens the chest.

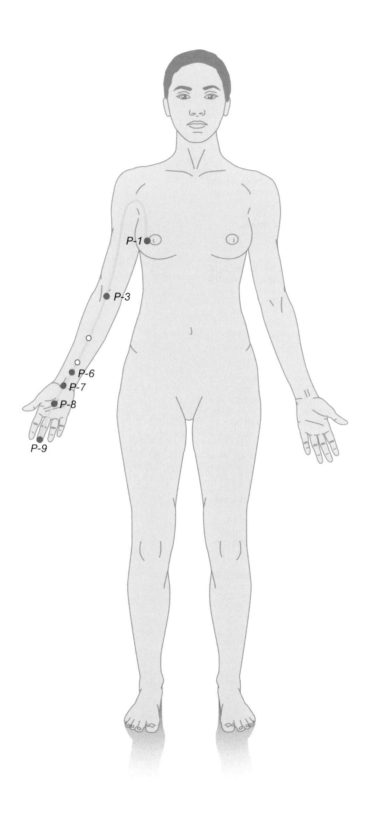

# The Triple Heater (Sanjiao) Channel

### SJ-1 Surge Gate

0.1 cun proximal to the corner of the base of the fourth fingernail on the ulnar side.
*Main Areas it Benefits:* Mind. Ears. Sanjiao channel.
*Main Functions:* Clears heat. Benefits the ears. Resuscitates consciousness.

### SJ-4 Yang Pool

On the dorsum of the wrist, between the ulna and carpal bones, in the depression between the tendons of extensor digitorum communis and extensor digiti minimi.
*Main Areas it Benefits:* Wrist. Sanjiao channel. Ears.
*Main Functions:* Tonifies Yuan qi. Regulates the Sanjiao.

### SJ-5 Outer Gate

Between the radius and ulna, 2 cun above SJ-4, on the radial edge of the extensor digitorum communis tendon, close to the radial border.
*Main Areas it Benefits:* Lungs. Liver. Ears. Head. Eyes. Forearm and wrist. Sanjiao channel.
*Main Functions:* Releases the exterior and dispels wind. Dispels stasis and smoothes the Liver. Clears interior and exterior heat. Descends excessive yang. Alleviates pain.

### SJ-10 Heavenly Well

1 cun proximal to the olecranon in the depression formed when the elbow is flexed.
*Main Areas it Benefits:* Elbow. Arm. Sanjiao channel.
*Main Functions:* Regulates qi and Blood. Alleviates pain and swelling.

### SJ-14 Shoulder Crevice

In the posterior depression below the ridge of the acromion when the arm is abducted. To aid location SJ-I4 is directly posterior to LI-15.
*Main Area it Benefits:* Shoulder.
*Main Functions:* Regulates qi and Blood. Alleviates pain and stiffness.

### SJ-17 Wind Screen

Behind the ear lobe, at the centre of the depression formed between the mastoid process and the mandibular ramus.
*Main Areas it Benefits:* Ears. Face. Throat. Neck.
*Main Functions:* Benefits the ear. Alleviates pain. Clears heat. Dispels wind. Treats the facial nerve.

### SJ-23 Silken Bamboo Hollow

In the depression at the lateral end of the eyebrow.
*Main Areas it Benefits:* Eyes. Temple.
*Main Functions:* Regulates qi and Blood and alleviates pain. Dispels wind and clears heat. Clears the eyes.

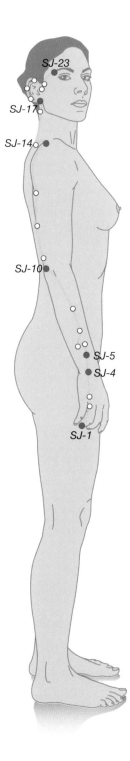

# The Gallbladder Channel

### GB-1 Pupil Bone Hole

In the hollow on the lateral margin of the orbit, approximately 0.5 cun lateral to the outer canthus.
*Main Areas it Benefits:* Eyes. Outer canthus.
*Main Functions:* Dispels wind and heat. Regulates qi and Blood. Benefits the eyes and vision.

### GB-12 Mastoid Process

In the depression inferior and posterior to the mastoid process.
*Main Areas it Benefits:* Ears. Back and sides of head.
*Main Functions:* Relaxes the body and calms the mind. Dissipates stasis. Alleviates pain.

### GB-14 Yang White

On the forehead, 1 cun above the midpoint of the eyebrow, directly above the pupil when the gaze is fixed straight ahead.
*Main Areas it Benefits:* Forehead. Eyes. Supraorbital area.
*Main Functions:* Calms the mind. Dispels wind and heat. Dispels stasis. Alleviates pain.

### GB-20 Wind Pool

Below the occiput, midway between Du-16 and the mastoid process, in the depression between the trapezius and sternocleidomastoid muscles.
*Main Areas it Benefits:* Head. Occiput. Neck. Eyes. Ears. Brain. Mind. Muscles. Entire body.
*Main Functions:* Relaxes the body. Descends rising yang. Benefits the Sea of Marrow.

### GB-21 Shoulder Well

On the top of the shoulder, midway between the spinous process of C7 and the tip of the acromion. On the highest point of the trapezius muscle.
*Main Areas it Benefits:* Neck. Shoulder. Upper back. Lungs. Chest. Breasts. Uterus. Head. Mind. Temple. Face. Eyes. Ears. Nose.
*Main Functions:* Strongly descends qi. Dispels stasis. Clears the chest. Induces menstruation and labour.

### GB-24 Sun and Moon

On the mammillary line, 4 cun lateral to the midline, in the seventh intercostal space. Inferior and slightly lateral to Liv-14.
*Main Areas it Benefits:* Hypochondrium. Ribs. Gallbladder. Chest. Epigastrium. Abdomen.
*Main Functions:* Spreads Gallbladder qi. Alleviates pain. Dispels dampness and heat.

### GB-25 Source Gate

On the lower back, at the free and of the twelfth rib.
*Main Areas it Benefits:* Kidneys. Lumbar area. Flank.
*Main Functions:* Benefits the Kidneys. Transforms dampness and heat. Regulates qi and blood. Alleviates pain.

### GB-30 Jumping Circle

On the postero-lateral aspect of the hip joint, one third of the distance between the prominence of the greater trochanter and the sacral hiatus, when the thigh is flexed.
*Main Areas it Benefits:* Thigh. Entire lower limb.
*Main Functions:* Dispels wind, cold and damp. Regulates qi and Blood. Alleviates pain.

### GB-34 Yang Mound Spring

In the depression anterior and inferior to the head of the fibula. Approximately 1 cun lateral and superior to St-36.
*Main Areas it Benefits:* Sinews. Joints. Flank. Hypochondrium. Gallbladder. Chest. *Main Functions:* Regulates qi. Dissipates stagnation. Alleviates pain. Benefits the sinews. Regulates the Gallbladder and Liver.

### GB-40 Mound Ruins

At the centre of the sizeable depression, anterior and inferior to the lateral malleolus.
*Main Areas it Benefits:* Ankle. Foot. Gallbladder. Mind. Emotions.
*Main Functions:* Regulates qi. Clears dampness and heat.

### GB-44 Foot Opening to Yin

0.1 cun proximal to the lateral corner of the base of the fourth toenail.
*Main Areas it Benefits:* Gallbladder channel. Head. Eyes. Mind.
*Main Functions:* Restores consciousness. Clears the head and brain. Benefits the eyes.

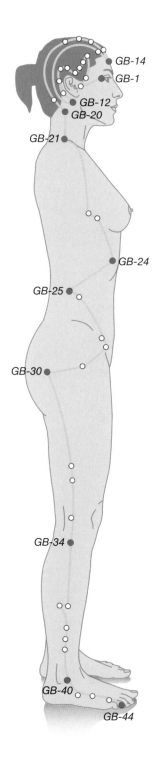

GB-14
GB-1
GB-12
GB-20
GB-21
GB-24
GB-25
GB-30
GB-34
GB-40
GB-44

# The Liver Channel

### Liv-1 Big Mound

0.1 cun proximal to the lateral corner of the base of the big toenail.
*Main Areas it Benefits:* Head. Nervous system. Uterus.
*Main Functions:* Subdues interior wind. Calms the mind. Arrests bleeding.

### Liv-3 Supreme Surge

On the dorsum of the foot, in the depression distal to the junction of the first and second metatarsal bones.
*Main Areas it Benefits:* Abdomen. Digestive and reproductive systems. Chest. Head. Eyes. Nervous system.
*Main Functions:* Circulates Liver qi and dispels stasis. Nourishes Yin and Blood. Cools the Liver. Regulates menstruation.

### Liv-4 Mound Centre

In the depression anterior to the prominence of the medial malleolus, medial to the tibialis anterior tendon, when the foot is at a right angle to the tibia.
*Main Areas it Benefits:* Ankle. Abdomen.
*Main Functions:* Spreads Liver qi. Harmonises the lower Jiao.

### Liv-5 Woodworm Channel

5 cun above the medial malleolus, in a small depression immediately posterior to the medial tibial border.
*Main Areas it Benefits:* Genitourinary system. Mind. Liver.
*Main Functions:* Spreads Liver qi. Benefits the genitals and uterus. Clears damp heat.

### Liv-8 Spring at the Bend

On or slightly proximal to the medial end of the transverse popliteal crease. About 1 cun anterior to Kd-10 when the knee is flexed.
*Main Areas it Benefits:* Lower Jiao. Genitals. Uterus.
*Main Functions:* Nourishes Blood and yin. Cools the Liver. Clears dampness and heat.

### Liv-13 Bright Gate

Below the free end of the eleventh rib.
*Main Areas it Benefits:* Abdomen. Hypochondrium. Chest. Digestive system.
*Main Functions:* Harmonises the Liver and Spleen. Boost Spleen qi.

### Liv-14 Qi Cycle Gate

On the mammillary line, 4 cun lateral to the midline, in the sixth intercostal space.
*Main Areas it Benefits:* Hypochondrium. Chest. Breast. Abdomen.
*Main Functions:* Spreads Liver qi. Dispels stasis. Cools Blood.

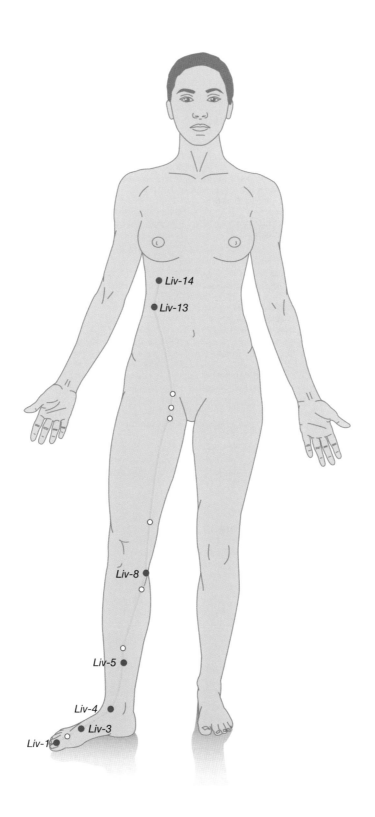

# The Ren Mai
# (Conception Vessel)

### Ren-1 Meeting of Yin

At the centre of the perineum, midway between the posterior border of the genitals and the anus.
*Main Areas it Benefits:* Genitals. Mind.
*Main Functions:* Boosts the lower Jiao. Lifts sinking qi. Increases libido.

### Ren-3 Central Pivot

On the anterior midline, 4 cun below the umbilicus. I cun superior to the pubic symphysis.
*Main Areas it Benefits:* Bladder. Uterus. Lower Jiao.
*Main Functions:* Dispels dampness, heat and cold. Strengthens the genitourinary system.

### Ren-4 Original Qi Gate

On the anterior midline, 3 cun below the umbilicus.
*Main Areas it Benefits:* Entire body. Abdomen. Small Intestine. Bladder. Uterus.
*Main Functions:* Augments Yuan qi. Nourishes yin and Blood. Calms the mind. Reinforces the Kidneys. Regulates qi and Blood. Strengthens the lower Jiao. Benefits the Small Intestine.

### Ren-5 Stone Gate

On the anterior midline, 2 cun below the umbilicus. I cun superior to the pubic symphysis.
*Main Areas it Benefits:* Abdomen. Uterus.
*Main Functions:* Mobilises Yuan qi. Warms and strengthens the lower Jiao.

### Ren-6 (Lower) Sea of Qi

On the anterior midline, 1.5 cun below the umbilicus.
*Main Areas it Benefits:* Entire body. Lower Jiao.
*Main Functions:* Tonifies and warms yang. Lifts sinking qi. Warms the abdomen. Regulates qi in the lower Jiao.

### Ren-8 Spirit Gateway

At the centre of the umbilicus.
*Main Areas it Benefits:* Umbilicus. Abdomen. Whole Body.
*Main Functions:* Tonifies, warms, lifts and revives yang. Regulates qi in the abdomen.

### Ren-12 Middle of the Stomach

On the anterior midline, 4 cun above the umbilicus.
*Main Areas it Benefits:* Stomach. Abdomen. Whole Body.
*Main Functions:* Tonifies the Stomach and Spleen. Harmonises the middle Jiao and descends rebellious qi. Nourishes fluids and yin. Dispels cold from the Stomach. Soothes the heart and calms the mind.

### Ren-14 Great Palace Gate

On the anterior midline, 6 cun above the umbilicus. This point may be just below or at the tip of the xiphoid process.
*Main Areas it Benefits:* Heart. Chest. Epigastrium.
*Main Functions:* Soothes the heart and calms the mind. Harmonises the Heart and Stomach.

### Ren-17 Chest Centre (Upper Sea of Qi)

At the centre of the chest, on the anterior midline, level with the fourth intercostal space, between the nipples.
*Main Areas it Benefits:* Heart. Lungs. Chest. Breast. Whole body.
*Main Functions:* Regulates qi and dispels stasis. Tonifies qi. Calms and balances the mind. Benefits the chest.

### Ren-22 Celestial Prominence

On the anterior midline, just superior to the suprasternal (jugular) notch.
*Main Area it Benefits:* Throat.
*Main Functions:* Descends rebellious qi. Alleviates cough.

### Ren-24 Sauce Receptacle

In the depression under the lower lip (at the midpoint of the mentolabial sulcus).
*Main Areas it Benefits:* Face. Teeth and gums. Eyes.
*Main Functions:* Treats disorders of the salivary glands, gums and teeth.

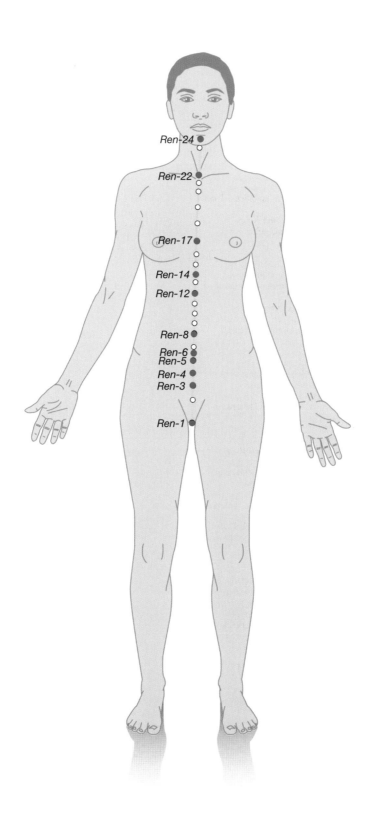

Ren-24
Ren-22
Ren-17
Ren-14
Ren-12
Ren-8
Ren-6
Ren-5
Ren-4
Ren-3
Ren-1

# The Du Mai (Governing Vessel)

### Du-1 Long Strong

Midway between the tip of the coccyx and the anus.
*Main Areas it Benefits:* Anus. Coccyx. Spine.
*Main Functions:* Benefits the anus and rectum. Regulates qi.
Benefits the spine.

### Du-2 Lumbar Point

On the posterior midline, at the sacrococcygeal hiatus.
*Main Areas it Benefits:* Sacrum. Coccyx. Lumbar spine.
*Main Functions:* Regulates qi and Blood. Alleviates pain.
Benefits the spine.

### Du-4 Life Gate

On the posterior midline, below the spinous process of L2.
*Main Areas it Benefits:* Lumbar area. Spine. Lower limbs.
Urogenital system. Uterus. Whole body.
*Main Functions:* Tonifies Kidney Jing and Kidney yang.
Dispels cold and dampness. Alleviates pain. Clears heat.
Benefits the lower Jiao and genitourinary system. Increases
fertility and vitality. Treats chronic diseases.

### Du-14 Large Vertebra

On the posterior midline, below the spinous process of C7.
*Main Areas it Benefits:* Lungs. Chest. Heart. Mind. Cervical
spine. Head.
*Main Functions:* Regulates ascending and descending of
Yang qi. Clears heat. Subdues internal wind. Releases the
exterior. Regulates qi and Blood. Benefits the spine.

### Du-16 Wind Palace

Directly below the external occipital protuberance.
*Main Areas it Benefits:* Head. Brain. Sense organs. Spine.
*Main Functions:* Dissipates wind. Regulates qi and Blood.
Alleviates stiffness and pain. Clears the sense organs. Relaxes
the body and calms the mind. Balances the nervous system.

### Du-20 Hundred Convergences

At the midpoint of the line connecting the apexes of both ears.
*Main Areas it Benefits:* Head. Sense organs. Rectum. Uterus.
Whole body.
*Main Functions:* Descends excessive yang and subdues wind.
Lifts sinking qi. Clears the head and sense organs. Calms the
mind.

### Du-26 Man Centre

Above the upper lip on the midline, approximately one third
of the distance between the bottom of the nose and the top of
the lip.
*Main Areas it Benefits:* Mind. Nose. Face. Spine.
*Main Functions:* Benefits the nose. Clears the face and eyes.
Restores consciousness and stimulates the mind. Regulates qi
and Blood and alleviates lumbar pain.

### Du-28 Gum Intersection

Inside the mouth, on the frenulum at the junction of the upper
lip and gum.
*Main Areas it Benefits:* Gums. Mouth. Nose.
*Main Functions:* Benefits the gums. Clears heat.

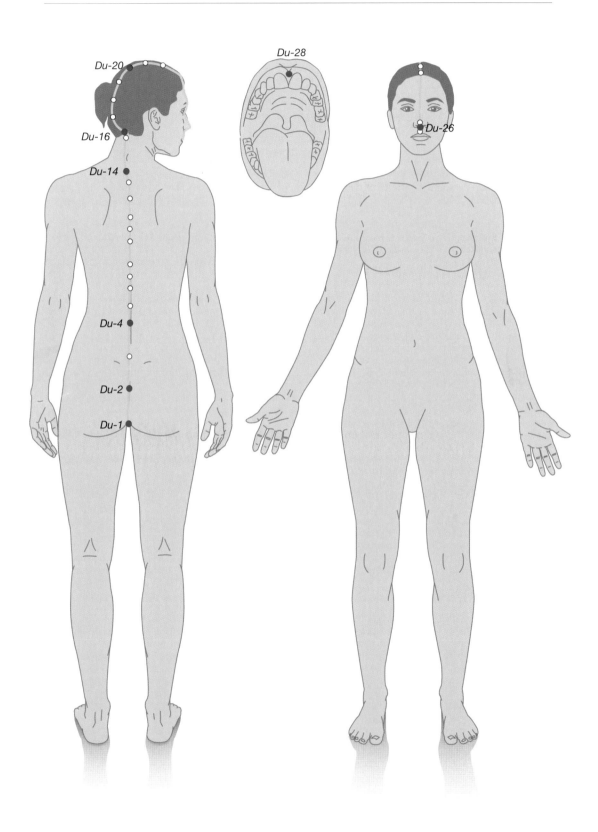

# Overview of Traditional Oriental Bodywork

The blanket term for traditional Chinese bodywork is *An Mo* (*Anma* or *Amma* in Japanese). An Mo literally means Press (An) and Rub (Mo), which is a somewhat inadequate title because a wide variety of techniques and principles are involved. An Mo has four major branches, each one defined by the specialised techniques which characterise it and the particular role it plays within the Chinese medical system. The four branches of An Mo are: 1. General massage (Pu Tong An Mo); 2. Push-Grab method (Tui Na An Mo); 3. Cavity Press method (Dian Xue An Mo); and 4. Ki method (Qi An Mo).

### General massage (Pu Tong An Mo)

Pu Tong An Mo is generally referred to simply as *An Mo* (or *Anma* in Japan). It is for relieving muscular soreness, generally smoothing blood and Ki circulation and for relaxation. It requires no detailed knowledge of Ki channels or Oriental medicine theory. In China and Japan, plus some other oriental countries, many of the practitioners are blind. This is because blind people cannot see the receiver's undressed body, so that in the older, more puritanical societies, there was less embarrassment when being massaged by them. Massage was also one of the easiest ways for a blind person to earn a living within cities of the orient.

The core technique of Pu Tong An Mo is similar to the 'muscle kneading' technique practised by practitioners of Swedish massage. In Pu Tong An Mo, this technique is called *Grabbing the Dragon* (Zhua Long). "Dragon" in this context refers to the muscles or tendons. The aim of this form of massage is to relax body and mind, to allow Ki and blood to circulate smoothly, and to remove the aches and pains caused by an accumulation of waste products in the muscles after hard exercise. Mostly however, it is used as a means of enjoyment.

### Push-Grab method (Tui Na An Mo)

Tui Na An Mo is usually just called *Tui Na*. It is named according to its two basic technique categories: Tui (push) and Na (grab to control). Tui Na has two distinct branches: one is for treating injuries such as bruising and injuries to ligaments, tendons, joints and bones; the other is for treating specific illnesses. Because it is used for treatment rather than relaxation, it requires a sound understanding of Oriental medicine principles.

Tui Na for injuries is commonly practised within the field of martial arts, where such injuries are common. In this context it is called Fall Strike method (Die Da) to reflect its martial arts application. This type of Tui Na developed from a system of bone and joint realignment that was practised by physicians during the Song dynasty (960–1126 A.D.) and throughout the Ming dynasty (1368–1644 A.D.).

Tui Na for illness is often used instead of acupuncture in situations where needling is difficult (such as with children, who tend to move and therefore bend or break the needles), or where the recipient is 'needle shy'; although it is also commonly used alongside acupuncture. For this reason, it is has been used extensively in the treatment of young children at least since the beginning of the Ming dynasty (1368 A.D.).

Tui Na is becoming increasingly popular outside the orient due to a more liberal attitude by the Chinese towards researching, reasserting and disseminating their heritage of traditional medicine.

### Cavity Press method (Dian Xue An Mo)

Dian Xue literally means, *point cavity*; so this method of bodywork focuses on stimulating acupressure points (*tsubo* in Japanese). The pressure used in Dian Xue is more direct and penetrating than that used in Tui Na, which focuses more on the soft tissues. Therefore, Dian Xue can be viewed as the main precursor of shiatsu, although aspects of Tui Na and particularly Qi An Mo (described below) also contributed. Very little written material is available on the history of Dian Xue. Oral dialogue given from generation to generation suggests that it was first initiated by Southern style and internal style martial artists and later fully developed by physicians.

In China today, many Tui Na practitioners are also versed in Dian Xue, so it is not uncommon to find Point Cavity Push-Grab (Dian Xue Tui Na) practitioners.

### Ki method (Qi An Mo)

Ki method is the art of transferring or transmitting Ki from the giver to the receiver. It is also known as *Curing with External Ki* (Wai Qi Liao Fa).

Ki method is divided into two categories; one involving direct body contact and the other involving no direct body contact. The body contact method is further sub-divided into a *Ki projection method* and a *Ki resonance method*. Ki projection method is used to supplement acupressure techniques (Dian Xue) insofar as the physician will project their own Ki into the acupressure point to nourish deficient Ki or remove excess Ki. Ki resonance method involves the practitioner lightly touching the receiver's skin to allow their Ki to correspond with, or 'resonate' with the receiver's Ki. Many shiatsu practitioners in both the East and the West are currently exploring methods akin to these.

The non-contact Ki method is very similar to the Ki resonance method except that the practitioner does not actually make contact with the body. They will hold their fingertips or the palm of their hand a few inches away from the receiver and direct Ki towards or away from specific areas of their body. It is what we would recognise these days as Qigong healing.

# Chronology of Bodywork Development in China and Japan

**8000 B.C.**
CHINA: Stone needles found at Neolithic sites in China.

**2550 B.C.** (approximately)
CHINA: Estimated date of writing of the oldest detailed resource on Oriental medicine: *The Huang Ti Nei Jing Su Wen*, believed to have been written by the legendary Yellow Emperor, Huang Ti.

**2205–1766 B.C.** (Xia dynasty)
CHINA: Acupuncture develops using stone, bone and thorns.[1.]

**1766–1122 B.C.** (Shang dynasty)
CHINA: Stone and bone acupuncture needles replaced by bronze. Inscriptions reveal that different illnesses were already named according to problems generated from organs.[2.]

**1122–206 B.C.** (Zhou and Qing dynasty)
CHINA: Internal and external treatments recorded for cuts, swellings and broken bones.[3.]
CHINA: Records of epilepsy treated with bodywork.[4.]
CHINA: First reference to Yin and Yang given in the *Yi Jing* (*Book of Changes*), written around 700 B.C.[5.]
CHINA: First reference to Five Elements appears during the Warring States Period of 476–221 B.C.[5.]
CHINA: Yin/Yang and Five Element theories merge between 340–260 B.C.[5.]

**206 B.C.–221 A.D.** (Han dynasty)
CHINA: The famous doctor Hua Tuo encourages the combining of acupuncture and bodywork (particularly massage and alignment techniques for dislocated and broken bones).[6.]
CHINA: The term 'An Mo' first appears in a written text which quotes its existence in texts of an earlier period, including the *The Huang Ti Nei Jing Su Wen* (*Yellow Emperor's Classic of Internal Medicine*); implying it is established practice in an earlier period.[7.]
CHINA: First mention of bodywork used for emergency first aid.[8.]
CHINA: First description of massage given with the feet (now a popular shiatsu style!).[9.]
CHINA: Techniques akin to the acupressure component of modern day shiatsu are mentioned in ancient text.[10.]

**265–420 A.D.** (Jin dynasty)
CHINA: Bodywork methods for correcting dislocations, addressing swelling and pain, and reviving from unconsciousness become well documented.[11.]
JAPAN: Korean immigrants brought Chinese medicine and culture to Japan in the 5th Century A.D. Korean doctors and scholars were invited to Japan to share their knowledge with the Japanese in the 6th Century A.D.[12.]

**605–618 A.D.** (Sui dynasty)
CHINA: Records show that An Mo physicians had become firmly established as part of the Imperial Hospital staff.[13.]
CHINA: Self-applied bodywork (akin to do-in) taught widely.[14.]
JAPAN: In 608 A.D. Prince Shotuku sent Japanese students to China to learn Chinese medicine and culture. Japanese priests and scholars go to China throughout the 7th Century A.D. to copy and bring back medical texts.[15.]

**618–907 A.D.** (Tang dynasty)
CHINA: Records of official medical posts were kept, detailing those who were *Doctors* or *Masters* of An Mo.[16.]
CHINA: Records show that there were more An Mo practitioners and students than acupuncturists and herbalists working in the Imperial Hospital at that time.[17.]
CHINA: Comprehensive bodywork systems are described in detailed texts, such as Lao Zi's, *49 Bodywork Techniques*.[18.]
CHINA: Bodywork techniques applied to the abdomen first documented.[19.]
JAPAN: Bodywork methods exported to Japan between 742–756 A.D., (the ancestors of Japanese anma and shiatsu).[20.]
JAPAN: Oriental medicine in Japan begins to follow an independent course from China, from the mid 9th Century A.D.[21.]

**960–1206 A.D.** (Song dynasty)
CHINA: First description of the role of bodywork to facilitate childbirth.[22.]
JAPAN: The first Japanese medical text, called *Ishimpo*, compiled in 984 A.D.[23.]
CHINA: Clear guidelines about when to use stationary pressure (a hallmark of modern day zen shiatsu) and when to use moving or rubbing techniques are clearly documented.[24.]

JAPAN: Renewed influence on Japanese medicine from Chinese mainland, due to renewed trade with China (after 300 years of relative isolation). During this period, the influence of court physicians diminished in favour of Buddhist monks, who played a key role in importing and adapting Chinese medical knowledge.[25.]

**1206–1368 A.D.** (Yuan dynasty)
CHINA: Tui Na An Mo bodywork prescriptions compiled.[26.]

**1368–1644 A.D.** (Ming dynasty)
CHINA: Tui Na emerges as a primary treatment for small children.[27. 28. 29.]
JAPAN: Three different approaches to medicine emerged in Japan between the 16th and 17th Centuries: The Gosei school – based on contemporary Chinese medical thought and development of the era; The Koho school – adhering to older traditional Chinese medical teachings; and the Rampo school – influenced by Western medicine.[30.]

**1644–1911 A.D.** (Qing dynasty)
CHINA: Bodywork treatment of skeletal injuries formulated into eight technique categories: Mo (touch), Jie (connect or 'connection'), Duan (hold up or 'support'), Ti (lift), Tui (push), Na (grab), An (press or 'apply pressure'), and Mo (rub).[31.]
CHINA: Countless books on bodywork published in 18th and 19th Centuries as Tui Na spreads amongst lay society.[32.]
JAPAN: Western medicine ideas and practice entered Japan as the result of trading with the Dutch during the Edo period (1602–1868 A.D.).[33.]
JAPAN: A monk called Mubunsai developed treatments applied solely through the abdomen (hara).[33.] This abdominal bodywork method became known as *Ampuku*, and was further developed as a particular application for gynaecological problems and childbirth. In 1765 the use of ampuku techniques in obstetrics was described in the book *San-Ron* (the *Description of Birth*) by Dr. Sigen Kangawa.
JAPAN: The blind acupuncturist 'Sugiyama' introduced uniquely Japanese innovations to acupuncture application and established Oriental medical schools for the blind during the early Edo period.[33.]
JAPAN: The ruling Shoguns reject the European influences exposed to Japan via the Dutch and Portuguese and encouraged the development of oriental traditions.

JAPAN: The Shoguns decreed that anma was a profession that could be practised by blind people (because of their enhanced sense of touch resulting from their lack of sight). However, due to their lack of sight, blind people had less educational opportunities, resulting in the decline of the medical aspects of anma, thus causing it to be given more for relaxation and pleasure than for treatment.
JAPAN: 1868 (period known as the *Meiji Restoration*), new government resolves to modernize Japan and later requires all physicians to pass an exam in Western medicine. Then a system of occupational training in acupuncture and bodywork is established for the visually impaired.[34.]

**1911 A.D. to the end of 20th Century**
CHINA: Bodywork methods used by martial artists revealed to lay society; particularly from the Shaolin and Wudang schools of bodywork, predominantly consisting of acupressure methods (i.e. *Cavity Press* or *Dian Xue An Mo*).[35.]
JAPAN: 1918: Acupuncturists in Japan can only obtain a licence to practice by following a revised list of acupuncture points which bare no resemblance to traditional channels or points, but are arbitrarily arranged according to a grid system.[36.] (Bodywork therapists of that time are generally influenced to follow this lead – *author*).
JAPAN: 1919: A book called *Shiatsu Ho* was written by Tamai Tempaku, which is the first time the word shiatsu seems to have appeared in print. Tempaku practised anma, ampuku and do-in. He also studied Western anatomy and physiology, and Western massage methods. His work influenced other practitioners to advance the development of shiatsu towards its modern form.
JAPAN: 1925: Tokujiro Namikoshi, who at first intuitively practised anma on his mother to help relieve her arthritis, studied bodywork and opened the Shiatsu Institute of Therapy in Hokkaido.[37.]
JAPAN: 1939: A society is formed for the intensive study of the Classics, eventually leading to the restoration of classical channels and points (tsubos).[38.]
JAPAN: 1940: Tokujiro Namikoshi moved his centre to Tokyo, establishing the Japan Shiatsu Institute. However, Namikoshi used the Western medical model as a theoretical basis rather than re-establishing classical theory, channels and tsubos.[37.]
JAPAN: After WW2, the U.S. occupying forces under General McArthur attempted to ban all traditional Oriental medicine in Japan in the belief that they were unscientific and unsanitary practices. A sustained legal

battle by Oriental medicine practitioners resulted in a new law passed in 1948 that guaranteed the right to practice traditional forms of medicine; although the western scientific influence has still predominated, leaving those who work Ki channels and use classical theory still a minority group within Japan.

JAPAN: 1955: Shiatsu is legally registered as part of anma, but to the frustration of shiatsu practitioners, not officially considered independent of anma.[37.]

JAPAN: 1957: Namikoshi's now renamed Japan Shiatsu School was officially licensed by the minister of health and welfare.[37.]

JAPAN: 1964: Shiatsu is finally recognised as a distinct therapy, separate from anma.[37.]

JAPAN: 1974: Tokujiro Namikoshi published details of his shiatsu method in his book, *Shiatsu Therapy: Theory and Practice.*

JAPAN: 1976: Katsusuke Serizawa produced *Tsubo: Vital Points for Oriental Therapy.* Serizawa was awarded a Doctor of Medicine degree in 1961 in recognition of his scientific work to prove the location and efficacy of the tsubos found along Ki channels. His work pioneered much of today's acupressure methodology; especially the use of devices such as electronic 'tsubo stimulators'.

JAPAN: 1977: Shizuto Masunaga produced the book *Zen Shiatsu*, which is the name given to the style of shiatsu pioneered by him. Through his book and through his Western and Japanese students, Masunaga subsequently influenced the practice and development of shiatsu in the West. Masunaga emphasised the use of an extended system of Ki channels that have come to be known as the zen shiatsu meridians. He also developed his own method of diagnosis through touching or viewing areas on the hara and back. In addition, he formulated a concise hypothesis for a unique shiatsu diagnosis / treatment model, distilled from traditional Oriental medicine, his clinical experience and his knowledge of psychology.

JAPAN: 1981: Shizuto Masunaga dies, but his successors and other practitioners continue to develop shiatsu, both in Japan and throughout the West.

## 21st Century

CHINA, JAPAN, THE WEST: Scholars and practitioners of Oriental medicine enter an era of re-evaluating and re-interpreting classical Oriental medicine theory as more source material is discovered or revealed by China.

# References

1.  *The Foundation of the Chinese Medicine in Category of Bone Injury*, by Ding Ji-Hua and Wu Chengde. Taipei, Taiwan. 1986.
•   This work quotes comments recorded in *Shan Hai Jing, Dong Shan Jing* (Mountain Ocean Classic, East Mountain Classic) and *Shuo Wen Jie Zi* (Analysis of documents with *Explanation of Terms*) by Xu Shen.
2.  The *Jia Gu Wen* (*Oracle Bone Scripture*) discovered during an archaeological dig at a Shang dynasty burial ground, consists of 160,000 pieces of turtle shell and animal bone covered with inscriptions detailing different sicknesses in relation to organ dysfunction.
3.  *Li Ji, Yue Ling Meng Qiu.*
4.  As recorded in the *Shi Ji* (*Historical Record*), the famous doctor Bian Que asked his assistant Zi You to massage Prince Guo, who suffered from epilepsy.
5.  *Science and Civilization in China*, Vol. **2**, by Joseph Needham, Cambridge University Press. 1956.
6.  Also, Dr. Zhang Ji-Zuo, in his book, *Shang Han Ran Bing Lun* (*The Theory of Typhus – Contamination*) summarised Oriental medical theory and treatment strategies and recorded many methods of bodywork treatment.
7.  *The Completeness of An Mo*, by Xiao Wen-Zhong. Taipei, Taiwan. 1986.
•   This work quotes from a commentary made during the Han dynasty (*Han Shu Yi Wen Zhi – Han's Book of Art and Scholarship*), on the oldest Chinese medical text, the *Huang Di Nei Jing* (*Yellow Emperor's Classic of Internal Medicine*) which mentions that "*during the reign of the Yellow Emperor, Qi Bo had written ten classics of An Mo ..*". Unfortunately these ten classics have been lost. Also, in a sub-section of the *Huang Di Nei Jing*, called the *Su Wen* (in the specific chapter on Blood, Qi, Shape and Spirit), conditions of numbness are fully described in relation to their treatment with bodywork and herbs.
8.  *The Refined Collection of An Mo Tui Na Techniques*, by Li Mao-Lin. Beijing, China. 1985.
•   This work quotes Dr Zhang Zhong-Jing in his book from the Han dynasty, *Jin Kui Yao Lue* (*Prescriptions from the Golden Chamber*), where he wrote, "*Use the hand to press on the chest, and move frequently*", as a prescription for attempting to revive someone who has been hanged.
9.  *The Completeness of An Mo*, by Xiao Wen-Zhong. Taipei, Taiwan. 1986.
•   This work quotes from a commentary made during the Han dynasty, *Yi Fa Fang Yi Lun* (*Treatise on Different Methods of Proper Treatment*), where it says: "*In the central region (of China), there are millions of living things in the heaven and earth, because the land is flat and wet. Thus, the food eaten by the people is varied and those people do not like to work. Therefore, the illnesses are mainly paralysis and withering, cold and hot. They should be cured by leading (the Qi) with An (An Mo) and Qiao. When people are inactive, their bodies become inactive and weak. They are therefore subject to illness caused by rapid changes in the weather. Their condition can be improved by enhancing their Qi circulation through An (An Mo) and Jiao (i.e., using the feet to massage)*".
10. *Ling Shu Jing* (*Spiritual Axis*). Beijing. 1981. First published in 100 B.C.
•   In Chapter 51, page 381, it says: "*If you want to get the points or examine them, you have to rub them. Inside (the point), there will be some reaction or pain; ...*".
•   In Chapter 75, page 544, it says: "*First, attentively observe and differentiate the fullness or emptiness of the channels by pressing with the fingers, using sliding techniques, and also rubbing and flicking the points*".
11. *The Refined Collection of An Mo Tui Na Techniques*, by Li Mao-Lin. Beijing, China. 1985.
•   This work quotes comments recorded in book from the Jin dynasty, *Shi Hou Jiu Zu Fang* (*The Methods of Preparing for Emergencies; Reviving from Unconsciousness*) by Dr. Ge Hong, where it says: "*To revive from a sudden faint,...., use the fingers to grab Renzhong cavity (a tsubo located just below the nose), which will immediately revive the patient*".
•   This work quotes comments recorded in another document from the Han dynasty by Dr. Ge Hong, *Bao Pu Zi*. It says: "*Where*

*there is swelling and pain, using the hands to massage can cure*".

12. *Introduction to Meridian Therapy*, by Shudo Denmai. Tokyo. 1993. Seattle. 1990, pp. 1–2.
13. *Sui Shu Bai Guan Zhi* (*The Record Of Hundreds of Officers in the Sui dynasty*). An original text.
• This work recorded that there was a division of an mo within the Imperial Hospital, led by two An Mo physicians.
14. *The Completeness of An Mo*, by Xiao Wen-Zhong. Taipei, Taiwan. 1986.
• This work quotes comments recorded in book from the Sui dynasty, *Zhu Bing Yuan Hou Lun* (*Thesis on the Origins and Symptoms of Various Diseases*) by Dr. Chao Yuan-Fang, where it says that self-massage for healing was taught in various places.
15. *Introduction to Meridian Therapy*, by Shudo Denmai, Tokyo. 1993. Seattle. 1990.
• Page 2. Here it states that the Japanese Government sent priests and scholars to the capital of China in the 7th Century, to study, where they copied many medical texts and brought them back to Japan.
16. *Tang Shu Zhi Guan Zhi* (*Record of Official Positions in the Tang Dynasty*). An original document; older and newer editions.
• These works recorded the names of men who were Masters of An Mo. The newer edition records a medical division which had one Doctor of An Mo and four Masters of An Mo.
17. *Tang Liu Dian* (*Tang's Six Records*). An original document.
• This work recorded that there were 56 An Mo technicians and 15 An Mo students in the Imperial Hospital; more than the number of acupuncturists and herbalists.
18. *Qian Jin Fang* (*Thousand Gold Prescriptions*) by Dr. Sun Shi-Mao. An original book from the Tang dynasty.
• In this book, Dr. Sun Shi-Mao introduced the 49 Bodywork Techniques of Lao Zi.
19. *The Refined Collection of An Mo Tui Na Techniques*, by Li Mao-Lin. Beijing, China. 1985.
• This work quotes comments recorded in a book from the Tang dynasty, Wai Tai Mi Yao (The Extra Important Secret), by Dr. Wang Tao, who writes: "*Rub both hands to make them warm, use them to massage the stomach; (this is) able to lead Qi downward*".
20. *The Completeness of An Mo*, by Xiao Wen-Zhong. Taipei, Taiwan. 1986.
21. *Introduction to Meridian Therapy*, by Shudo Denmai. Tokyo. 1993. Seattle. 1990, page 2.
22. *The Refined Collection of An Mo Tui Na Techniques*, by Li Mao-Lin. Beijing, China. 1985.
• This work quotes extracts from a book written during the Song dynasty, *Yi Shuo* (*Talks on Medicine*), by Dr. Zhang Ben.
• Dr. Zhang Ben quotes a talk given by Dr. Pan An-Shi on how to use massage to help in childbirth.
23. *Introduction to Meridian Therapy*, by Shudo Denmai. Tokyo. 1993. Seattle. 1990.
• Page 2 mentions Japan's first medical text, *Ishimpo*, by Tamba Yasunari, published in 984 A.D.
24. *The Refined Collection of An Mo Tui Na Techniques*, by Li Mao-Lin. Beijing, China. 1985.
• This work quotes extracts from the fourth volume of the archived records written during the Song dynasty, known as, *Jing Ji Zong Lun* (*The Total Record of Economics*). In this volume it says: "*(for some sicknesses) you can use An (press), (..for others you can use Mo (rub). Together, this is An Mo. When Mo (rub) do not An (press). Use herbs sometimes. These are An and Mo. Fit (them) to the right purpose*".
25. *Introduction to Meridian Therapy*, by Shudo Denmai. Tokyo. 1993. Seattle. 1990.
• Page 2. Denmai describes how the collapse of the stable social order of Japan, based on control by the imperial family, during the 12th Century A.D. led to the war lords assuming control and promoting trade with China. This led to renewed Chinese influence exerting a strong influence on the practice of medicine in Japan.
26. *Shi Yi De Xiao Fang* (*Effective Prescriptions of Well Known Doctors*), by Dr. Wei Yi-Lin. An original document.
• Dr. Wei Yi-Lin systematically compiled effective Tui Na and other bodywork prescriptions discovered before the Yuan dynasty. The Yuan dynasty was particularly abundant in written records concerning bodywork methods for realigning and setting

bones; the most well known from this period being, *Yong Lei Qian Fang* (*Permanent Seal Techniques*), by Dr. Li Zhong-Nan. In fact "bone correction Tui Na" was listed as the "thirteenth category" in the medical system.
27. *The Refined Collection of An Mo Tui Na Techniques*, by Li Mao-Lin. Beijing, China. 1985.
• This work quotes extracts from books written during the Ming dynasty, *Xiao Er An Mo Jing* (*Bodywork Classic for Small Children*) and *Xiaou Er Tui Na Mi Jue* (*The Secret of Tui Na for Small Children*), by Dr. Zhou Yu-Fu. Also, the appendix of *Zhen Jiu Da Cheng* (*The Great Compendium of Acupuncture and Moxibustion*), written in 1601 A.D., by Dr. Yang Ji-Zhou, contained a section called *Bao Ying Shen Shu An Mo Jing* (*The Classic of Marvellous Bodywork Massage Techniques for Protecting Babies*), which discussed the use of bodywork to treat illness in babies.
28. *The Completeness of An Mo*, by Xiao Wen-Zhong. Taipei, Taiwan. 1986.
• This work quotes from the book written during the Ming dynasty, *Xiao Er Tui Na Fang Mai Huo Ying Mi Zhi Quan Shu* (*The Complete Book of Secret Keys to Massaging Small Children*), which added much knowledge to the field of infant bodywork.
29. *Guide to Infantile Tuina*, by Gong Yunlin. 1604. An original text.
• This work offers a systematic illustrated guide to bodywork for infants; describing infantile diseases in rhymed songs.
30. *Introduction to Meridian Therapy*, by Shudo Denmai. Tokyo. 1993. Seattle. 1990.
• Page 3, states that the Gosei, Koho and Rampo schools each contended with and influenced each other until the end of the 19th Century.
31. *Yi Zong Jin Jian; Zheng Gu Xin Fa Yao Zhi* (*The Gold Study of Medicine; The Important Keys to Correcting Bones*), by Dr. Cheng Qian. An original text.
This work systematically compiled all of the publications on the subject of bodywork, and became the authority on the treatment of injuries.
32. *The Completeness of An Mo*, by Xiao Wen-Zhong. Taipei, Taiwan. 1986.
• This work quotes from many books written during the Qing dynasty, such as, *Tui Na Guang Yi* (*The Wide Definition of Tui Na*), by Dr. Xiong Ying-Xiong, *You Ke Tie Jing* (*The Iron Mirror for Small Children*), by Xia Yu-Zhu; and, *You Ke Tui Na Mi Shu* (*The Secret Book of Infantile Tui Na*), by Dr. Luo Qian-An.
33. *Introduction to Meridian Therapy*, by Shudo Denmai. Tokyo. 1993. Seattle. 1990.
• Page 3 reveals that Dutch physicians influenced major schools of Japanese medicine, particularly the school founded by Ishizaka Sotetsu, so that they became based on a more accurate knowledge of anatomy.
34. *Introduction to Meridian Therapy*, by Shudo Denmai. Tokyo. 1993. Seattle. 1990.
• Page 4 reveals that tight government control over the practice of healing arts in Japan, leads to the government controlling the only avenue for formal education in Oriental medicine. In 1911, Japanese acupuncturists are for the first time, required to obtain a licence to practice from the government.
35. *Chinese Qigong Massage – General Massage*, by Dr. Yang Jwing-Ming.
36. *Introduction to Meridian Therapy*, by Shudo Denmai. Tokyo. 1993. Seattle. 1990.
• Page 4. Denmai describes that many practitioners in Japan resented this interference by the government, which stimulated a fervent revival of research into classical texts.
37. *The Complete Book of Shiatsu Therapy*, by Toru Namikoshi. Japan Publications. 1981, page 21.
38. *Introduction to Meridian Therapy*, by Shudo Denmai. Tokyo. 1993. Seattle. 1990.
• Pages 6–7, describes how acupuncturists Okabe, Inoue and colleagues formulate a system of treatment strategies based on the *Nan Jing Jiao Shi* (*Classic of Difficulties*), first published in 100 A.D. They called this system *Meridian Therapy* because it restored the channels (meridians) to the central focus.